SPATOPIA

SPAtopia

Unique Spa Experiences from around the Globe

by Amy Rosen

Copy-Editor: Lloyd Davis
Design: Andrew Roberts
Printer: Transcontinental

Library and Archives Canada Cataloguing in Publication

Rosen, Amy
    SPAtopia : unique spa experiences from around the globe / Amy Rosen.

Based on the author's World of Wellbeing columns in *The Globe and Mail*.
ISBN 1-55002-528-7

    1. Health resorts—Guidebooks. I. Title.

RA794.R68 2004   613'.122   C2004-903713-7

1   2   3   4   5   08   07   06   05   04

 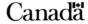

Conseil des Arts du Canada   Canada Council for the Arts   Canada   ONTARIO ARTS COUNCIL CONSEIL DES ARTS DE L'ONTARIO

We acknowledge the support of the **Canada Council for the Arts** and the **Ontario Arts Council** for our publishing program. We also acknowledge the financial support of the **Government of Canada** through the **Book Publishing Industry Development Program** and **The Association for the Export of Canadian Books**, and the **Government of Ontario** through the **Ontario Book Publishers Tax Credit program**, and the **Ontario Media Development Corporation's Ontario Book Initiative**.

Care has been taken to trace the ownership of copyright material used in this book. The author and the publisher welcome any information enabling them to rectify any references or credits in subsequent editions.

J. Kirk Howard, President

Photographs used in this book courtesy of Fairmont Hotels and Resorts, Four Seasons Hotels and Resorts, Haldimand Hills Spa Village, Stillwater Spa, and Stoweflake Mountain Resort and Spa.

Cover photograph: Las Ventanas Al Paraiso, San Jose Del Cabo, Mexico. Courtesy of Rosewood Hotels & Resorts.

Printed and bound in Canada
Printed on recycled paper
www.dundurn.com

Dundurn Press
8 Market Street
Suite 200
Toronto, Ontario, Canada
M5E 1M6

Gazelle Book Services Limited
White Cross Mills
Hightown, Lancaster, England
LA1 4X5

Dundurn Press
2250 Military Road
Tonawanda, NY
U.S.A. 14150

SPAtopia

TABLE OF CONTENTS

Introduction 8

Spas in Canada

Silk Road Natural Spa, Victoria 12
The Spa at the Wedgewood Hotel, Vancouver 16
Skoah, Vancouver 20
Eveline Charles Salon & Spa, Vancouver 24
Ancient Cedars Spa at the Wickaninnish Inn, Tofino 28
The Spa at the Hotel Vancouver, Vancouver 32
Stillwater Spa, Calgary 36
Institut de Santé, Calgary 40
Elmspa, Toronto 44
The Chakra Spa, Toronto 48
The Spa at White Oaks Resort, Niagara-on-the-Lake 52
The Hillcrest Spa, Port Hope 56
Haldimand Hills Spa Village, Grafton 62
Le Spa, Hotel le St-James, Montreal 68
Ovarium Floatation Baths, Montreal 72
Bliss the Spa, Halifax 76
Spirit Spa, Halifax 80
Other Canadian Destination Spas 85

Spas in the United States

Regent Beverly Wilshire, Beverly Hills 88
The Spa at the St. Regis, Los Angeles 92
The Ritz-Carlton Huntington Hotel and Spa, Pasadena 96
Las Vegas Spas 100
Spa at the Four Seasons Resort, Dallas 104
The Spa at the Crescent, Dallas 110

The Spa at the Four Seasons Hotel, Chicago 114
The Fairmont Turnberry Isle Resort & Club, Aventura 118
Doral Golf Resort & Spa, Miami 122
The Spa at the Mandarin Oriental, Miami 127
Nemacolin Woodlands Resort & Spa, Farmington 132
Golden Orchid Spa, Frederick 136
Capital City Club and Spa, Washington, D.C. 140
The Spa at the Four Seasons Hotel, Philadelphia 144
3000BC Spa, Philadelphia 148
Elizabeth Arden Red Door Salon & Spa, New York 152
Affinia Fitness Spa, New York 156
Avon Salon and Spa, New York 160
Topnotch, Stowe 164
Stoweflake, Stowe 168

International Spas

Clinica Internacional, Cuba 176
Sandals Royal Bahamian Resort and Spa, Bahamas 180
Spas of Ocho Rios, Jamaica 186
Spa at the Four Seasons Resort, Uruguay 190
Hammam Majorelle, Morocco 194
Hof Weissbad, Switzerland 198
Spa Hopping in Switzerland 203

Airport Spas

208

Spas for Seniors

214

INTRODUCTION

Come on in. Relax. The spa-ing's fine…

The twenty-first century is shaping up to be quite a bit more stressful than previously anticipated. Little wonder, then, that spa-going has become one of North America's favourite new pastimes. Which is precisely why you need this book. Nary a week goes by without a splashy spa opening or the creation of some groundbreaking therapy, and it's all good news for people in search of new ways to unwind.

But where to go? What to do? What's going to happen to me once I get there? That's where *SPAtopia* comes in. Consider this your handy guide to stress busting and renewal, whether you're a spa newbie or seasoned pro. Here you'll find the inspiration that will lead to rejuvenation (and perhaps a bit of perspiration) by finding your own perfect spa haven.

From the opulent and sexy to the therapeutic and scary, you'll get the essence of a wide range of spas and treatments, location, design, clientele, service, food — and the bottom line on why you should go there. Handy contact information is also included so that you can immediately book your very own cold-fusion energy facial or Ayurvedic holistic body treatment.

As a Canadian girl with a taste for the good life, but an equal love of the more organic experiences off the beaten path, I'm here to cut through the clutter, to guide and to nurture you. But don't expect the regular spa roundup. This snappy little primer isn't about the twenty-five best Asian spas, the fifty most luxurious spas, or even how to set up a home spa. Those books have already been written. *SPAtopia* is different, in part, because I've spent the past year and a half circling the globe, visiting more than sixty spas in order to guide you from a firsthand perspective through a cross-section of spa society, from high-end retreats and brand new day spas to wellness centres and even a centuries-old public bathhouse (if you dare).

SPAtopia covers everything from vinotherapy treatments in Niagara-on-the-Lake to the old world elegance of a five-star health hotel in Switzerland, from the best spa treatments for seniors to a roundup of airport spas. Brimming with humour and bursting with detailed information, this is your personal introduction to the best in spas and their treatments, from Montreal to Jamaica and all points in between.

Spas are the hottest destination for the busy traveller looking to decompress. If you've bought this book, congratulations: you've taken a giant step towards a healthier, happier you.

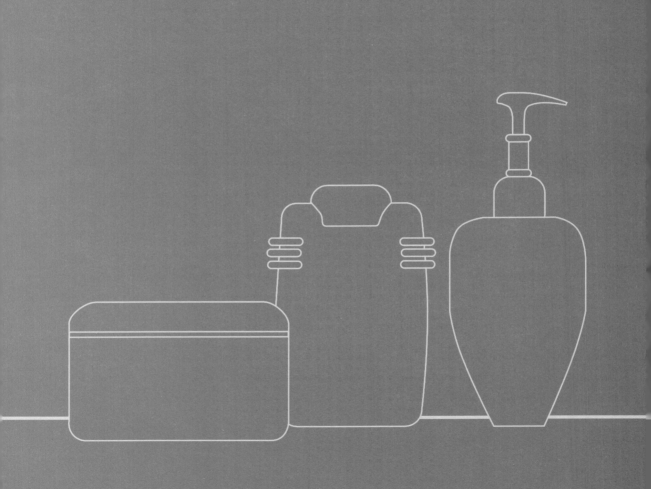

SPAS IN CANADA

SILK ROAD NATURAL SPA, VICTORIA

Long ago there was a trading route that spanned the Chinese empire, over which caravans carried sumptuous silks to the western edges of the region. Silk was an important commodity, so nomadic Central Asian tribes routinely attacked the caravans in hopes of capturing the traders' treasure. But then Chang Ch'ien, a wise Chinese explorer, got the idea of expanding the route to include these lesser tribes in the silk trade. Thus, the ancient Silk Road was born.

The geographic passage grew and prospered with the rise of the Roman Empire and, much later, found a new outpost on the shores of Victoria. "We're introducing Chinese culture and design into our area," says Silk Road co-owner Daniela Cubelic.

Think antioxidant green tea body wraps, fresh ginger exfoliation massages — and ancient Chinese secrets.

LOCATION

Victoria is a city built for wandering. Take an impromptu tour of the B.C. Legislature with its mural-clad rotundas, stained glass windows and rich, woodsy legislative chamber. Government Street is a spot for buskers, postcard shops, tartan clothing and an inordinate number of fleecewear shops. Silk Road, also on Government Street, is in the heart of Canada's oldest Chinatown, home to Tai Sang Company, Choi Hung Video, Peking House, oodles of noodle houses and pagoda-style telephone booths. The Silk Road storefront has floor-to-ceiling picture windows with views of cherry blossoms and Chinese lanterns.

DESIGN

The shop has a decidedly Asian-influenced décor with its flashes of vibrant Chinese red and warm putty, and black distressed floor. Rustic display tables and rows of open shelves bow under the strain of Mercury Retro teapots, Yixing pottery, botanical mists and glass jars filled with natural products like Silk Road Chai aromatherapy salts. Exposed brick and high ceilings carry on to the backroom tea bar that serves up and sells canisters of premium-quality loose teas from around the globe. Taking the creaky staircase down a flight, the three treatment rooms are warm and simple, done in bronzed brick and Japanese paper accents.

CLIENTELE

Tourists and locals alike come to browse and buy amidst this chic and unique retail experience. And since the spa treatments are all-natural, with an emphasis on wellness and relaxation (as opposed to the more cosmetic aesthetics offered elsewhere), the spa holds quite a strong appeal for men.

TREATMENTS

Silk Road offers a veritable teacart of natural aromatherapy spa experiences, like green tea facials, ginger-and-green-tea exfoliation massages, and tea-infused pedicures. Spa packages range from ninety minutes to the four-hour Aphrodite. Three-and-a-half-hour Bride and Groom packages include facials, manicures, aromatherapy massages and body wraps and cost just CDN$149 each.

The events calendar also features workshops on home spa treatments, how to plan a foolproof seduction, cooking with tea, and in-store Japanese tea ceremonies. In other words, everything you need to pamper yourself from head to toe. But the spa is perhaps best known for its foot pampering, like the Peppermint Pedicure, meant to renew and revitalize tired tootsies. You start by sitting in a chair and soaking your feet in a basin filled with warm water, mineral and sea salts, chamomile tea, essential oils and some river rocks for fiddling. Then your feet are dried and you lie down on the cozy massage table and fall asleep, if you're so inclined. Meanwhile, nails are cut, shaped and buffed, cuticles are trimmed, and feet are massaged with minty oils and spritzed with herbaceous tonics. The Silk Road does not believe in nail polish, so all fingers and toes have a natural finish. It's actually amazing how sexy healthy nails can look without further adornment.

SERVICE

A sip of smoky gunpowder green tea is offered to all who enter to shop or spa. And if you sidle up to the tea bar at the back, the knowledgeable staff will find the perfect blend to suit your needs through questioning and tasting. Heading down the stairs to the spa sanctuary, Jacquie is as quietly soothing as a mug of sweet tea on a Sunday afternoon.

BOTTOM LINE

Many spas boast modern, gender-neutral spaces, but most offer a mere handful of men's treatments. Not so at Silk Road. The roster includes men's pedicures and manicures, Mark Antony's Facial, the deluxe Adonis Facial and a goodly choice of guy-friendly wraps, scrubs and packages. With no fuchsia nail polish in sight, and the added bonuses of all-natural products, pottery and tea leaves to be bought and sipped, this place is bound to be just about anyone's cuppa.

INFORMATION

Silk Road. 1624 Government Street, Victoria, BC. Phone: (250) 704-2688.
Web: http://www.silkroadtea.com.
The Peppermint Pedicure lasts one hour and costs $35. Tea parties, ceremonies, tastings and workshops range in price from free to $45.

THE SPA AT THE WEDGEWOOD HOTEL, VANCOUVER

magine you're a downtown boutique hotel, rich with European elegance. You house a city-favourite restaurant and freshly reno-vated suites, and have recently earned an avalanche of industry awards, including *Travel + Leisure* magazine's Gold List, *Condé Nast Traveler's* Best Hotel in Canada, and *Vancouver* magazine's Best Bar & Lounge five years running. What's your next move? Launching a luxurious day spa, of course.

LOCATION

The Wedgewood is as centrally located as they come, in the heart of downtown Vancouver amidst galleries and museums, great shopping and dining, and equidistant from Stanley Park, English Bay and False Creek.

DESIGN

Many of the eighty-three rooms and suites have just been renovated and redecorated and are charmingly cozy in earth tones and accents of burnished bronze and black. The bathrooms feature Italian marble. The lobby is ultra-elegant, decorated with old world antiques and a crackling fireplace. The brand new (as of June 2003) second-floor spa is petite and deluxe (two treatment rooms, a smart little mirrored gym, steam and showers) with tumbled marble, walls of wood, wrought iron and fresh flowers.

CLIENTELE

The Wedgewood is considered one of the world's best business boutique hotels, so the majority of the guests are industry folk, many of whom visit the spa for everything from sports massages to the Executive Escape. In-room massage is also available and popular with the stressed-out bigwigs. Locals and visiting celebs that frequent Bacchus (Rod Stewart had dined there the previous evening) are also discovering the spa.

TREATMENTS

Hotel and spa owner Eleni Skalbania has chosen the Epicuren Discovery skin treatment system — "voted best overall prestige skin care line by *InStyle* magazine" — as the skin care line of choice for her spa's signature treatments, which include the

SPATOPIA

Cinnamon Enzyme Facial and the Ultimate Body Toning Treatment. The info blurb for the latter says it's specifically designed to target certain areas (such as limbs, stomach, neck and buttocks) and includes the use of enzyme cellulite cream and thermal body sculptural masks. It's meant to reduce puffiness and cellulite by lifting and smoothing slight dimpling. It promises immediate results, and the effects are said to last for a week. Sold!

This service begins, like most, with the subject naked and facedown on a massage bed. A rosemary lave, which cleanses and aids in circulation, is applied and wiped off, then the cellulite cream is massaged in (this contains caffeine, which draws out excess water from bloated bits). In addition, an orange lotion is also applied to stimulate and draw out toxins. Then things get weird. To assist in the absorption of the enzyme cellulite cream, open-weave gauze is applied to the targeted body parts, atop which the thermal body sculptural mask, which is rich in calcium, vitamins and minerals, is spackled. Heat builds up, in goes the good stuff and out comes the bad. After about twenty minutes it peels off like a cast. Enjoyable hot towel massages of the hands, feet and scalp are administered throughout, and after the casts are peeled off, mask residue is wiped away and a finishing application of cellulite cream is smoothed on, along with spritzes of orange blossom tonic. Verdict? It may only be wishful thinking, but I swear I could see a marked difference.

SERVICE

One of the reasons the Wedgewood is such an award winner is because of its impeccable service, which can no doubt be attributed to its guest-to-staff ratio of seven to one. Oh, *and* the fact that they leave freshly baked cookies by the bed at turndown.

FOOD & DRINK

The exceptionally handsome Bacchus is where chic scenesters come for the city's smartest cocktail hour, but it's also packed at lunchtime (the Wedgewood is right across from the Vancouver Court House), dinner and weekend afternoon tea. The menu is full of exciting French-influenced local delights, such as pan-roasted halibut with Dungeness crab and potato cake, crisped chorizo sausage and apple-tomato relish. With its plush banquettes, curvaceous bar and flattering lighting, it is little wonder that this spot is routinely voted the best romantic restaurant in the city. At the spa, lunch (or afternoon tea on weekends) is included in the price of all treatments running ninety minutes or longer, and you may take your meal before or after your spa experience, either in the treatment room or, better still, on the deck. Sensible spa options include the likes of a West Coast seafood platter with a young greens and chervil salad, and a seasonal fruit plate with yogurt or cottage cheese.

BOTTOM LINE

This is the little privately owned boutique hotel that could. The Wedgewood has won legions of loyal clients through its decadent interiors, delicious restaurant, excellent service and brand new spa. But if we're really being honest here, it gets my vote because I can now bounce a nickel off of my butt.

INFORMATION

The Wedgewood Hotel. 845 Hornby Street, Vancouver, BC. Phone: 1-800-663-0666. Direct line to the spa: (604) 608-5340. Web: http://www.wedgewoodhotel.com. The Ultimate Body Toning Treatment lasts 90 minutes and costs CDN$225, including spa lunch. Accommodations at the hotel start at $300 per night.

SPATOPIA

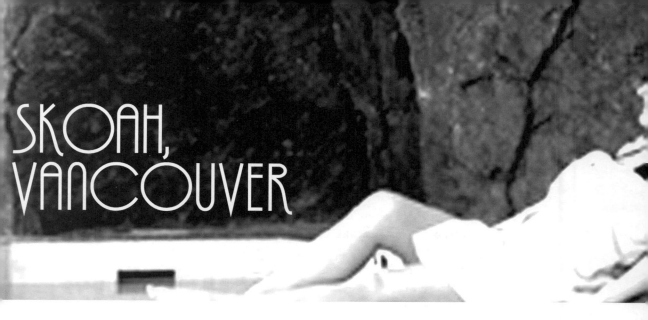

SKOAH, VANCOUVER

The concept of working out to stay young — getting that heart pumping, toning those muscles and following a sensible diet — is nothing new. But what about a training regimen for the skin?

After listening to feedback from customers at her burgeoning Yaletown spa, co-owner Andrea Scott realized that everyone was talking up its facials. "It was a calculated risk, but we decided to ditch the bikini waxing and pedicures and go skin [care] whole hog," she says. "After all, you don't go to Starbucks for a burger."

What Skoah came up with was the concept of "personal training for your skin." Here's how it works: the aesthetician gives you a facial, after which, like a personal trainer, she fills you in on your skin "workout program." Then you "train" at home with the new line of Skoah products, whose all-natural ingredients are the equivalent of your skin's healthy diet.

As it turns out, some workouts are an absolute pleasure.

LOCATION

Yaletown's distinctive brick-clad loading docks and warehouses have been gentrified over the past decade into contemporary lighting shops, home and apparel boutiques, cigar bars, a soup spot touting low-carb options, coffee houses (*bien sûr*), a Mini car dealership, galleries, oyster bars, spray-on tanning salons, a yoga centre, cosmetic dentistry clinics and oodles of glassy condos. Basically, if you were to draw up an imaginary blueprint for a utopian yuppie village, Yaletown would be it. It's also just off the False Creek Seawall between Expo 86's Science World and the Granville Street Bridge — so both downtown Vancouver and Granville Island are easily walkable.

DESIGN

Skoah boasts an airy, modern vibe that says "boutique hotel" more than downtown day spa. The walls are a light pistachio hue with blue accents and mahogany-look wood. There's tile work, track lighting and cork floors, plus exposed ductwork and whitewashed concrete that hearken back to the location's past life as a factory. The six treatment rooms, including one double room for skin-loving couples, are expansive and lovely with wood-trimmed mirrors, clean lines, cozy chairs, suspended sinks and cheery blue paint. Cool tunes — no Enya or waterfowl sounds here — pipe from the sound system.

CLIENTELE

A Facialiscious treatment (coupled with a night at the neighbouring new Opus hotel) was one of the gifts offered to all Oscar presenters this year, but aside from the glitterati most of the customers are young, hip, urban professionals in the 24 to 45 age range, a goodly 30 percent of whom are gents.

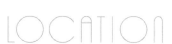

SPATOPIA

22

TREATMENTS

It starts with a welcoming bottle of Skoah water (other nice touches include a jar of Dubble Bubble gum in the bathroom and a free Lip Love balm when you leave). You get undressed, cozy up under the sheets and the personalized Facialiscious "workout" begins. It includes cleansing and toning, a gentle exfoliation with a gel that is 10 percent vitamin C and 2 percent AHA gel and which brings about a slightly prickly feeling. No steaming or scrubbing is needed after the gel's natural sloughing power has done its job. Then there's a peel made from things like grapes and apples; some extractions; a calming mask to take down the redness and add moisture; plus massages for the legs, face, hands and shoulders throughout.

Essentially, my workout started with getting clean and toned, then getting physical and getting treated, and ended with getting hydrated and protected. If I were to buy some of the products for home training sessions, they would include the likes of Tonik (with soothing arnica), Face Skotian (with blend of extracts from eleven plants) and Hydradew Mask (with kelp alginate).

Skoah offers only seven different treatments, from the Two Scoops of Skoah and Melted Muscles Massage to Facialiscious Sunny-Side Down (kind of like a facial for your back).

On a personal note, during the week following my Facialiscious workout, no fewer than five different people commented on how good my skin looked. And that almost never happens.

SERVICE

Decked out in a chic, pale-blue Skoah T-shirt and form-fitting pants, Laura-with-the-perfect-skin dishes out cucumber tonic, melon masks and mimosa massages with calmness and clarity. Then she polishes you off with a matte-look moisturizer so you can immediately show off your new visage in Yaletown without risk of your reputation being impugned. "Enjoy your Skoah gloah!" she says as you stride out the door.

BOTTOM LINE

On first blush, placing all your eggs in one skin care basket might seem a risky venture. But if that basket happens to be a gorgeous spa done up in modern hues, and those eggs are the best skin care treatments in their milieu, it doesn't seem so risky anymore. And when you add a fresh line of products with which to follow up at home, suddenly it sounds awfully smart.

INFORMATION

Skoah. 1011 Hamilton Street, Vancouver, BC. Phone: (604) 669-9775.
Web: http://www.skoah.com. (You can also buy Skoah products online at that address.) Prices start at CDN$15 and top out at $75. The Facialiscious treatment lasts about an hour and costs $90.

SPATOPIA

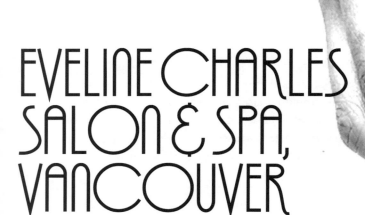

EVELINE CHARLES SALON & SPA, VANCOUVER

Some people know spas. Some people know business. And then there's Eveline Charles. She's the woman behind the eponymous spa and salon chain where Westerners in Calgary, Edmonton and more recently Vancouver have been enjoying cutting-edge hair design and the best in body and skin care for close to a decade. With an eye for detail and a head for commerce, Charles recently became the first woman to be inducted into the Alberta Business Hall of Fame, and was also voted Marketer of the Year by *Alberta Venture* magazine. Not bad for a small-town girl from northern Alberta. And now she's gearing up to take on the East.

LOCATION

The Vancouver spa sits on a busy corner in the South Granville neighbourhood, where you can take in the theatre of life from the great walls of second-storey picture windows: a guy runs for the bus in the rain; a couple walks hand in hand while drinking vente Starbucks coffees — in the rain. It's quite the happening strip, where old-moneyed dowagers co-mingle with young, über-hip fashionistas. Anchor stores Restoration Hardware and Caban mix with higher-end boutiques. There are especially good pickings in the discerning home décor shops and gourmet coffee houses. A couple of blocks down the street (between 12th and 14th avenues) sits a popular area for aficionados of English and Continental antiquing.

DESIGN

The two-storey spa has a gleaming retail shop selling Eveline Charles and Darphin products on the ground level. The second floor is expansive, expensive-looking and sleek, but contemporary touches such as sandblasted glass and oversized Martha Sturdy accent pieces warm it up, as do the textured cream-on-cream walls, a big fireplace, chocolate-brown African wood and bamboo touches. Think streamlined exotica.

   With four facial rooms, three massage rooms, two Vichy showers, a hydrotherapy tub, heated, vibrating-pedicure thrones and a long row of salon chairs, all propped up against those large picture windows, even on a gloomy day, it's cheery here.

CLIENTELE

Many are transplanted Calgarians thrilled that their hometown favourite is finally in Lotusland. There's also a mix of well-to-do's and bargain hunters who have all embraced the excellent spa treatments at lower-than-the-norm prices.

SPATOPIA

26

TREATMENTS

This is no middling midtown day spa: hand and foot care, men's facials, floral baths, hot stone massages, hair services — they do it all, and they do it all well. But since this is a salon and spa, let's start by getting a fresh new hairdo.

Ashley Harrison isn't only the artistic director of Eveline Charles, he's also a Contessa Award winner as best hairstylist in Alberta. He'll size you up, listen to your concerns and then go at you with the scissors. An hour or so later, you've had a mini-makeover (in this case, a chic mod cut with thick bangs), which makes extra sense here since Harrison was featured on an episode of TLC's *A Makeover Story*, to happy-tears results.

Now, how about some fancy feet to go along with that newly coiffed 'do? Once you've been cozily wrapped in a terry-lined, champagne-coloured robe, Angela begins the Eveline Charles Signature Pedicure by cranking the massage throne up to full torque as you kick back for a cooling foot spray. Then comes a warm foot soak. Toenails and cuticles get the once-over, rough spots are sanded down, feet are moisturized and an exfoliation treatment applied.

You get your choice of Eveline Charles' all-natural products, such as Mango Sugar and Coca-Nilla Scrub. Exfoliants range in degree of sloughing power from mild pomegranate and sesame seeds to full-strength citrus salt.

After the exfoliation comes a deep-leg massage, again with your choice of all-natural creams. (Tip: Go for the shea butter; it smells like butter-cream frosting). You finish off with a vitamin E–enriched paraffin treatment, which opens up the pores to help moisture penetrate, warms the feet and loosens the joints.

Finally, the polish goes on — all Eveline Charles colours, like sheer French Kiss pink — and everyone gets a mini-bottle of her chosen polish to take home. Nice touch.

SERVICE

The staff seem emotionally invested in both the place and the products, and can be counted on for an endless stream of helpful beauty tips. For example, what to do with coarse Semitic hair? "Use a paddle brush to straighten it and leave-in conditioner to smooth it," offers Ashley. They're talented and down-to-earth.

BOTTOM LINE

The all-natural products smell so good, you'll want to eat them. You leave with a brand new look, smelling like a bakery, and striding down Granville Street feeling like a frosted cupcake. And that's a good thing.

INFORMATION

Eveline Charles Salon & Spa. 1485 West 11th Avenue, Vancouver, BC.
Phone: (604) 678-5666.
In all, there are five locations across Canada. Haircuts are CDN$38–$75 for women, and $30–$55 for men. The Signature Pedicure lasts 90 minutes and costs $65.

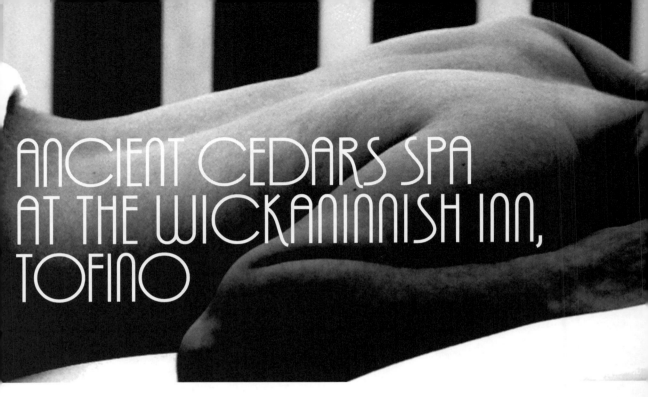

ANCIENT CEDARS SPA AT THE WICKANINNISH INN, TOFINO

Deep in the woods around Tofino, a few lucky souls are breathing deeply while sitting in Muskoka chairs overlooking Chesterman Beach. Their feet are soaking in large copper basins at Ancient Cedars Spa in the Wickaninnish Inn — the perfect setting for a high-end, laid-back West Coast spa vacation.

LOCATION

The Wickaninnish Inn is a gorgeous five-hour drive from Victoria. The scenery goes a little something like this: water, mountain, trees, water, mountain, trees. The inn is minutes from Tofino, where surf shops, good organic vittles and whale-watching tours are all at your disposal, and is located at the westernmost point of Chesterman Beach, at the gateway to Pacific Rim National Park Reserve and Clayoquot Sound.

DESIGN

The Ancient Cedars Spa looks a lot like the name sounds: the décor is loaded with rustic elegance in the form of cedar wood, stone and slate. There are five treatment rooms as well as manicure and pedicure stations. The nature-infused change rooms incorporate such touches as baskets full of Aveda products for pre- or post-treatment use, name cards on assigned wooden lockers, and tree branches as hooks for plush robes. Best is the front balcony — where you sit and luxuriate in foot soaks and ocean breezes — and the Cedar Sanctuary, a massage hut for two that includes floor-to-ceiling windows overlooking the Pacific, two massage tables and a fireplace.

CLIENTELE

The inn and spa don't come cheap, so expect to see wealthy Canadians and Americans (from Seattle), plus Hollywood types coasting in on private planes. Even with the addition of the new Wickaninnish-on-the-Beach, right next to the original lodge, you've still got to book suites six months to a year in advance.

TREATMENTS

If you've made the trip here, you might as well go whole hog and take in one of the spa's signature services, billed as "the best of earth and sea." One is the Sacred Sea Thalassotherapy treatment, a three-tiered process. First you're seated, clad in a robe, on a Muskoka chair in a little stone enclave on a deck overlooking the ocean, while you soak your feet in a large copper basin. At this point, you choose the Aveda essential oils and compositions that will be used during the treatment by first sniffing coffee beans to clear the olfactory palate. You narrow down the sixteen possible choices by smelling miniature bottles with names such as Earth Nature (to energize) and Full Spectrum (for grounding). Scents include orange and peppermint or geranium, lime and eucalyptus. Your selection made, a few drops of oil go into the foot bath and you kick back while the rooms are prepared.

The Sacred Sea treatment starts with a full-body exfoliation, using salts from the Dead Sea, infused with the oils you chose during the foot soak, as the medium. The scrub and hot-oil treatment isn't for the fragile, as it feels a lot like sandpaper, but the results are worth it.

Then you hop into the Bouvier hydrotherapy tub, where 144 jets, with the added impact of algae products and essential oils, massage the body in waves. Once you've towelled off, into a full aroma body wrap you go. The layering of foil, warm sheets and towels is lovely, and you smell of nature and sugar and spice. You also get a scalp and foot massage during this step. It finishes with a massage that uses Blue Oil, a balancing concentrate that wakes you up and lets you get on with your day.

SERVICE

Staff are young, cheery and West Coast casual — albeit dressed in black like so many Upper Canadians.

BOTTOM LINE

Ancient Cedars Spa uses natural products and treatments to totally mollify body and spirit in the wilds of the Pacific Rim. Couldn't be any better if Mother Nature had built it herself — and in a way, she did.

INFORMATION

Ancient Cedars Spa at the Wickaninnish Inn, Tofino, BC. Phone: 1-800-333-4604. Web: http://www.wickinn.com.
The Sacred Sea Thalassotherapy treatment is CDN$180 and lasts two hours.

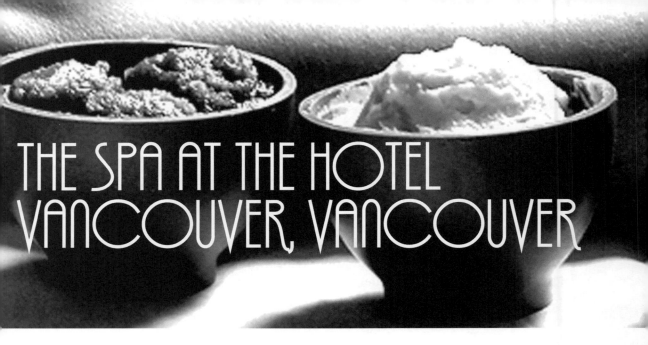

THE SPA AT THE HOTEL VANCOUVER, VANCOUVER

You've got to love Lotusland. Where else in Canada does the general populace think of wheatgrass shooters instead of B-52s when they imagine a night out? That said, there is little doubt that the relaxed inhabitants of this health-conscious city will outlive us all.

Sure, we can poke fun at their outdoorsy lifestyle, inordinate number of Starbucks franchises, the rainy winter weather and subsequent uniforms of Mountain Equipment Co-Op waterproof jackets. But Vancouver's natural beauty and temperate weather are part of what makes it a magnet for tourists. Perhaps in line with its philosophy of California-style healthy living, the city has an impressive repertoire of spas, including the Spa at the Hotel Vancouver, with luxurious treatments that are a steal for bargain-hunting massage addicts from south of the border.

LOCATION

There may be a Starbucks on every corner, but Vancouver's best lattes are actually available next to the Fairmont Hotel Vancouver at Café Artigiano. Beyond the easy access to a great caffeine jolt, there could not be a better place from which to explore the city proper. Nearby Stanley Park is available for biking or strolling, as is the sun-swept seawall. The Vancouver Art Gallery is right across the street, and Robson Street, the centre for shopping in Vancouver, is directly behind the hotel. The Pacific Centre (a three-block-wide mall) is also nearby. Take a twenty-minute walk to the south side of False Creek and English Bay and check out the public market at Granville Island, where you'll find organics, cut flowers, crafts and noshes. Many of these delectable products can be sampled at the city's myriad excellent restaurants, which feature Pacific Northwest cuisine based on regional ingredients from the land, sea and sky. It has been said that if Vancouver has a culture, it is dining out.

CLIENTELE

A steady stream of Alaskan cruise shippers, Washington state inhabitants, visiting Europeans and locals come and go for everything from wash and blow dries to pedicures and shiatsu massages.

SERVICE

Top-notch across the board.

SPATOPIA

DESIGN

The Fairmont Hotel Vancouver is an historic property that was refurbished in 1996 and is holding up in princely fashion. The imposing green copper roof of this 1939 château-style building dominates Vancouver's skyline, while the handsome lobby bar is packed nightly with martini-swilling vacationers enjoying live piano tunes and torch songs. Guest rooms have an air of prestige with their high ceilings, mahogany furniture and marble bathrooms. And then there's the subterranean spa. The reception area is lovely, with its wraparound dark-stained desk, hardwood floors, gold-leafed backdrop and walls stacked with shelves touting Kerstin Florian skin and body products from Switzerland.

But then things take a turn for the worse.

The Solace Spa group took over the spa in 1996 after the previous owner went bankrupt. Instead of completing renovations, the company basically slapped on a new coat of paint and bought a hamper full of towels. When I visited, the treatment rooms were marred by industrial rubberized flooring and outdated Formica counters. There was no ethereal relaxation room or cozy lounge area — amenities that regular day spa trippers have come to expect. It was a little surprising in a hotel of this size and stature.

Things, however, could be looking up. The facility has since been taken over by the Absolute Spa Group, who also operate the spa at Fairmont's hotel at the Vancouver airport (see page 208).

TREATMENTS

When a simple pedicure just won't cut it, book an indulgent three-hour spa package like the spa's Solace Soother. It begins with an hour-long massage of your choice: Swedish, aromatic, sports, shiatsu or reflexology. Try the sports massage with

Sherry; she'll work out knots and kinks you never knew you had. Next up is either a refresher facial, body wrap or body scrub (choices range from a Turkish scrub to an aromatic wrap). The thirty-minute refresher facial is so good, it puts its full-length counterparts to shame. It involves copious steps, including skin analysis, hot towels, black mud, exfoliation, lavender oil, intermittent spritzes of Neroli water, a finishing clarifying serum, moisturizer and eye cream. Then it's time to break for lunch: a massive plate of local and tropical fruit, plus a bowl of plain yogurt and slices of banana bread. The Solace Soother finishes off with either a shampoo and style in the salon or a paraffin manicure, which is one of the city's best. Three hours later, you leave the spa looking as clean and buffed as a six-year-old on her first day of school.

BOTTOM LINE

The location, staff, treatments and products are all impressive. The spa had everything going for it except for its small size and humdrum looks. An expansion or at least a face lift is deserved.

INFORMATION

The Spa at the Fairmont Hotel Vancouver. 900 West Georgia Street, Vancouver, BC. Phone: (604) 648-2909 or 1-877-684-2772. Web: http://www.fairmont.com. The Solace Soother was CDN$195 and lasted two and a half to three hours, including lunch. The hotel has 556 rooms, 42 suites, two restaurants, an indoor pool and health club.

SPATOPIA

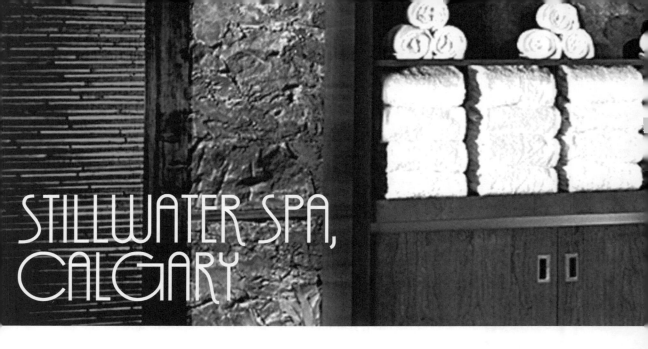

STILLWATER SPA, CALGARY

t's the little things in life that make all the difference: a firm hand-shake over a weak one; a full-on pratfall in lieu of a timid skid; chocolate with 70 percent cocoa, not 20.

At the new Stillwater Spa at the Hyatt Regency in Calgary, they've honed the little things to a fine art, which is why the Stillwater brand (two locations in Canada, seven worldwide) is making big waves in this competitive industry.

From the homemade granola bars in the change room to the refrigerated face cloths outside the steam room, spa-going out west has become as cultured, yet relaxed, as a picnic in your Sunday best.

DESIGN

The Stillwater Spa is located on the second floor of the Hyatt Regency Calgary, which three years ago gave a twenty-one-storey boost to the downtown skyline. The spa's décor sets the tone: warm wood, chocolate-coloured walls, chrome accents and splashes of jewel-toned fabrics. The treatment rooms feature original exposed stonework with rough-hewn framework. The spa lounge has a soothing waterfall wall and a burbling tropical-fish aquarium. The in-change room whirlpool is there for pre-treatment soaks, and a mini-fridge outside the steam room holds tiny containers of cucumber slices for puffy eyes, and moist towelettes for shvitzy faces.

AMBIANCE

Although this is a deluxe spa, the mood, in true Calgarian form, is casual. Women gabbing in the lounge over designer mineral water give it an air of upbeat serenity with a soupçon of downtown diva.

CLIENTELE

Working girls on a birthday binge, conventioneers with cash and locals who know a good thing when they see it.

SERVICE

Three names to remember: Christie, Carrie and Colleen. This "Triple C" is young, delightful and commendably certified.

TREATMENTS

The Kaolin Body Masque is a mixture of soft-clay powder blended with essential oils such as rose and lavender. It cleans, exfoliates, detoxifies and smoothes the skin like nobody's business. The application goes to work after you're wrapped in heated towels. During the gestation period, your face is treated to more warm towels dipped in herbed water, while the scalp gets a relaxing massage. Once you're unwrapped and showered, an all-over natural moisturizing massage completes the treatment.

The Deep Cleansing Facial rejuvenates and nourishes the skin, bringing it back into balance. All-natural products are used at the Stillwater, including plant-based cleansing milk, exfoliating peel, anti-aging apricot oil serum, purifying steam and custom-blended mineral mask. The deep foot massage is a definite bonus.

But sometimes all a gal really wants is some pretty polish on her nails. In that case, the spa manicure is a great pick-me-up, replete with a herbal hand soak that benefits from hot river stones and paraffin wax with rose oil. Begone, cruel hangnails. All nail colours are by manicurist to the stars Deborah Lippmann.

FOOD & DRINK

The food could be described as "typical with a twist" and includes such fare as organic chicken breast and sake-and-maple grilled prawns. What's more impressive is the wine list, most of the entries on which can be ordered by the glass. Catch — an upmarket seafood restaurant that was recently named the best new restaurant in Canada by *enRoute* magazine — is part of this high-end hotel and spa complex. Its oyster tastings and CanCon main dishes, including roasted East Coast lobster with beurre blanc, are beyond memorable.

THINGS TO DO

With cobblestoned Stephen Avenue Walk (a pedestrian mall) right out front, the Calgary Tower behind, and the Rockies just over yonder, how you spend your time here depends on the type of person you are.

Highbrow? The Glenbow Museum, Western Canada's premier exhibition of Native history and European settlement, is adjacent to the Hyatt Regency. Got a green thumb? Devonian Gardens, Alberta's largest indoor gardens, is a quirky refuge in the heart of the bustling downtown shopping district. Wild about warthogs? The Calgary Zoo is nearby, home to more than 900 cute and furry (and sometimes scary) creatures. And for all types, there's the Yodeling Sausage stand — offering "the best of the wurst" — just across the street.

BOTTOM LINE

With a frontier-chic clay body wrap, tasty spa vittles and a high-noon facial, any damsel who arrives in distress will ride off happily into the sunset.

INFORMATION

Stillwater Spa at the Hyatt Regency Calgary, 700 Centre Street. Calgary, AB.
Phone: (403) 537-4474. Web: http://www.stillwaterspa.com.
Hotel phone: (403) 717-1234; hotel Web: http://calgary.hyatt.com.
The Kaolin Body Masque is CDN$110, the Spa Manicure is $45 and the Deep Cleansing Facial is $99.

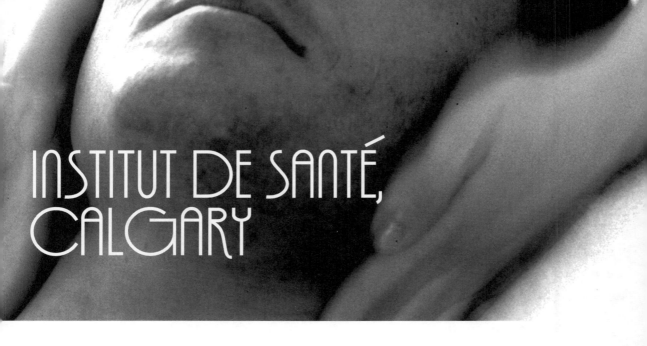

INSTITUT DE SANTÉ, CALGARY

We all know that beauty isn't skin deep. Sometimes you actually have to break through the epidermis and get right down to the muscle to get the results you're looking for. That's where Calgary's Institut de Santé comes in. Conceived and owned by Dr. Wendy Smeltzer (BSc, MD, CCFP, FCFP), this day spa offers the full spectrum of conventional services, but also goes one step further, performing such advanced medical skin treatments (read, performed only by a physician) as high-level chemical peels, Botox injections, microdermabrasion, soft-tissue augmentation and IPL (intense pulse light) photofacials.

LOCATION

This mocha brown, three-storey office building is set on Calgary's Fourth Street, a residential area with a bustling main drag of trendy shops, galleries and hipster hangouts.

DESIGN

For an office building, the institute is really quite classy. Each of the rooms — aesthetics, Vichy, massage, hydrotherapy, manicure and the doctor's room — is done up in soothing shades of caramel and cream, with accents of velvet, wood, frosted glass and wrought iron. Soothing spa music plays in the background and a subtle, fresh fragrance lingers. You'd never know what was happening behind some of these closed doors.

CLIENTELE

This is a sophisticated centre for skin rejuvenation, where qualified doctors and technicians treat the effects of sun damage, acne and aging. A large proportion of clients are baby boomers. But since it also offers some of the best body treatments, massages and gentlemen's services in town, it's anybody's game. Group spa nights and incentive packages are available, although it has yet to host a Botox party.

SERVICE

The front-of-the-house crew is dapper in basic black and snappy Burberry neckerchiefs. Doctors and aestheticians are top-notch, informative and friendly. Dr. Smeltzer's bright smile and twinkly eyes are as reassuring as they could be when she utters the words, "So, you feeling up for a chemical peel?"

TREATMENTS

The experience begins with a consultation with a physician. Dr. Smeltzer, the founder of Institut de Santé, is also a founding director of Spa Canada, a four-year-old association with ninety-one members that is setting national standards for spas from St. John's to Victoria.

In the doctor's room, you recline on a treatment chair as she surveys your face. "When looking at skin rejuvenation, you're looking at three layers," she explains. "The epidermis, which is the outer layer; the dermis, which is the thicker, more structured layer of the skin; and then the deep-muscle tissue underlying the skin."

Shining a bright light in your face, she makes you smile and frown repeatedly while you look in a mirror. No frown lines — good. Smile lines, yes, but not permanent. "You're a brow raiser — raise, relax, raise, relax… See? You get these lines every time you do that." (Note to self: Quit being such a brow raiser.)

After surveying the damage, the doctor decides that a 50 percent alpha-hydroxyl peel is in order. (They can go as high as 70 percent). This is a surface treatment that will speed up the skin's natural exfoliation process and plump up the layers underneath. It helps alleviate sun damage, slight acne scarring and other skin irregularities.

The doctor mixes up the alpha-hydroxyl solution, which is clear, thick and viscous, with not much of a scent. She brushes it on and sets a timer for three minutes while fanning your face for comfort. You feel a slight prickly sensation. After the timer bell rings, a neutralizing, moisturizing base gel goes on for five minutes to soothe the skin. The process is non-invasive — there's no scarring or scabbing — but you may look a bit flushed afterward. You'll see the results immediately — it's as if you're the new poster girl for Ivory.

It's recommended to adhere to home follow-up instructions and to repeat the peel two weeks later. A total of six treatments yields the best results.

The spa has undergone a large expansion to accommodate its new Living Better lifestyle programs — three-month-long plans to get clients started on making effective life changes. A team of highly-touted specialists, including personal trainers, a dietitian, psychologists and kinesiologists, will provide support to get you on the road to a new and improved you.

BOTTOM LINE

The Institut de Santé offers up herbal tea, a fresh face and significant lifestyle changes. It's a relaxing spa that gets results. Just what the doctor ordered.

INFORMATION

Institut de Santé. 508 24th Avenue SW, Calgary, AB. Phone: (403) 228-2772. Web: http://www.institutdesante.com.
A chemical peel costs CDN$80. A set of the recommended six treatments is $450. The price of the Living Better programs is determined by an assessment, but the average is $1,000 a month.

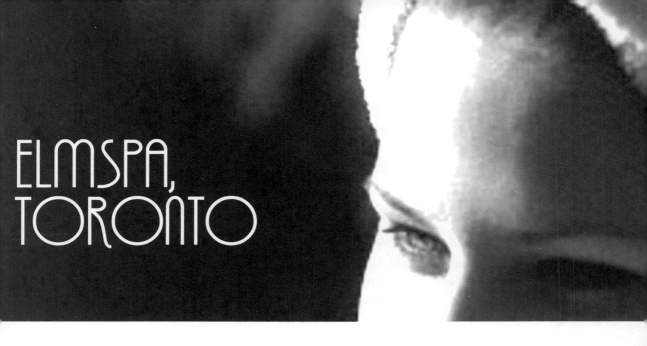

ELMSPA, TORONTO

Brought to you by the makers of that grand old dame, the Elmwood Spa (which celebrated its twentieth anniversary in 2002), Toronto's Elmspa is like the Elmwood's hip kid sister who has travelled the world and returned home toting a bunch of goodies in her backpack — and a Thai boyfriend with great taste.

The new high-end day spa is, in a word, urban, from its city-core locale and treatments with time-saving variations to its trend-setting good looks. It is also, in another word, refreshing, from the lemongrass iced tea to the cedar garden terrace and easy access to midday stress relief.

One additional, olfactory descriptor: herbaceous. The scent of herbs is in the air, in the treatments and in the products. And although it can be relaxing, woe is she with a heightened sense of smell.

LOCATION

The downtown intersection of Church and Wellesley is at the heart of Toronto's gay village, and a block south is where you'll find the squat, refurbished office building that houses the Elmspa. Hanging out on the steps in front of Second Cup is the perfect spot for people-watching (or gawking), especially during the Pride Parade each June. Nearby are the 519 Community Centre, Cawthra Park, and good eats at Byzantium and Inspire restaurants. The spa is also just blocks away from Cabbagetown, Riverdale and the haughty Bloor-Yorkville shopping district.

DESIGN

A strong Thai influence runs throughout, from the icy lemongrass tea to the music, décor and treatments. The look is born of nature, with a feng shui space plan and a Zen vibe. The perimeter of the spa is defined by a drenched-wood walkway (with a positive chi flow), anchored by river stones, linen window coverings and recessed water-bubble wall features.

Six treatment rooms bearing the names of indigenous Canadian trees (maple, pine) lie at the spa's core. Most of the wood is cherry-coloured Merbeau culled from a managed forest. It works especially well in the modern change rooms, in combination with white marble, sleek chrome finishes and salvaged-wood stools (made from timber brought up from the Pacific floor by B.C. divers).

The four-station manicure/pedicure area overlooks the expansive cedar deck terrace, handcrafted by All-Aboard Youth Ventures, a nonprofit organization that trains youth at risk. Come summertime, the spa plans to take its nail services outside and build a canopy for outdoor Thai massages. It also hopes to harvest herbs on the deck to be used in some signature treatments.

CLIENTELE

Patrons include Bloor Street shoppers and boardroom types looking for respite, area gents wanting to spruce up via sports pedicures and manly facials, and spa scenesters getting in on the ground level.

TREATMENTS

In the nineteenth century, a battalion of 400 women armed with spears guarded the king of Siam. They were said to perform drills better than their male counterparts, and were crack spear-throwers to boot. When they returned from their tour of duty they were often rewarded with a special back massage. Recognizing that life in downtown Toronto can sometimes feel like a battlefield, the Elmspa offers a treatment called the Siam Herbal Tension Release. The spine holds many nerve endings and meridian lines (or chi channels), so the Siam service concentrates primarily on the back. Part one of the fifty-minute treatment entails a ten-minute shvitz in the frosted-glass steam room. It's good and steamy, but the marble is clammy and cold, and the steam is forced through rocks covered with herbs, so it smells strongly of burning underbrush.

Now you're ready for step two, an herbaceous foot soak coupled with a shoulder and neck massage. After the soak, you lie facedown on a treatment table while an exfoliating scrub made from nutmeg and coriander seeds (among other things) is scrubbed into the back, then removed with warm towels. Hot cloth compresses containing lemongrass and eucalyptus are then used to massage the back, down to the lower lumbar vertebrae, in deep, twisting motions. The compresses open up the back and loosen tense muscles, and a good, oily aromatic massage finishes the deed. The stress falls away and you emerge smelling like a heaping plate of *aloo gobi* (with a side of cucumber *raita*).

More mainstream is the Elmspa facial, which cleanses, exfoliates and moisturizes using Swissline products, bringing your face back into kissing form after a particularly harsh winter. (How harsh was it? "My apartment was so dry," Leda says, "my cats were letting off sparks.")

SERVICE

Most of the aestheticians here are the best of the bunch from the Elmwood Spa and have signed on for the excitement of a burgeoning new venture in dishy new digs. (Hint: ask for the excellent Leda.) Considering that the new campus of Elmcrest College for massage therapy (established in 1976) shares the floor with the Elmspa, it's a good guess that some graduates will be making their way over to the spa soon.

BOTTOM LINE

This is a downtown day spa where time seems to slip through an hourglass instead of flashing by on a digital clock. Unwind in the steam room for ten minutes and allow a body mask to sink in for ten more. True relaxation takes time, so let the spa do its thing. Even though the location is in the midst of city hustle and bustle, if you visit when you're in a rush, you're missing the point.

INFORMATION

Elmspa. 557 Church Street. Phone: (416) 964-4500. Web: http://www.elmspa.ca. The Siam Herbal Tension Release for the back is CDN$129 (it is also available for the full body, which takes 80 minutes, or just the legs, clocking in at 40 minutes). The 50-minute Elmspa facial is $96.

SPATOPIA

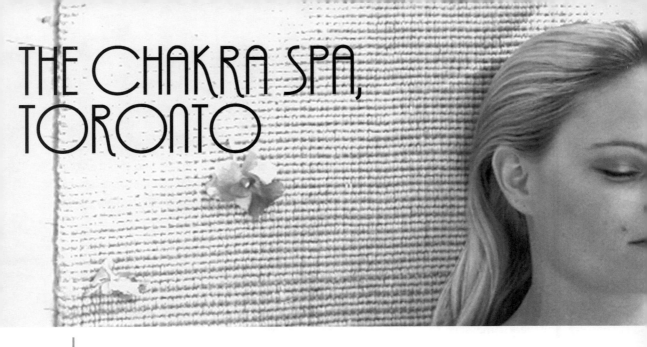

THE CHAKRA SPA, TORONTO

f you're feeling the urge to dig a bit deeper — as in "inner psyche" deeper — than medical science and long-held Western beliefs allow, it might be time to investigate a kind of spa therapy that requires both cleansing breaths and a leap of faith.

The premise behind Toronto's Chakra Spa is that before you can heal yourself you must connect with your physical, emotional and spiritual sides, thereby treating the whole being, rather than just the knot in your back.

Chakra is a Sanskrit word that means "wheel." It refers to the seven energy centres that control our consciousness and energy systems. These chakras are supposed to function as valves that regulate the body's energy flow and reflect decisions we make during the daily grind. It's an Indian philosophy that's all about balance, relaxation, healing — and brightly coloured lights.

LOCATION

The strip of Eglinton Avenue between Bathurst Street and Strathearn Road has a bit of a Yiddish soul. It resembles a Lilliputian village replete with synagogues, a kosher butcher, Montreal bagels, the Jerusalem Restaurant and that favourite Jewish pastime, Chinese food. Near the end of this stretch, a short distance from the Allen Road turnoff, is the Chakra Spa. It is a happy sanctuary within the chaos of the city, although even the classical music, ambient nature sounds and tinkling water features don't completely block out the roar of rush-hour traffic.

DESIGN

About a year ago, the Natural Choice day spa went through a renovation, a name change and an extensive shift in philosophy and emerged as the Chakra Spa. The new space is warm and inviting, done up in vibrant hues of oranges, pinks and blues.

Upon entering, you are hit by a scent that's an intoxicating mix of spicy and sweet. This freebie aromatherapy hit changes daily. From the wind chimes and bamboo water fountain to the brocade armchairs, the slippers and even the mixed berry tea, everything has been carefully calculated by spa founder Lisa Julien to welcome and ready you for what lies ahead.

CLIENTELE

This spa is mostly a she-thing: 95 percent of the clients are women, many of whom are stressed-out soccer moms trying to reconnect with their inner Earth Mothers.

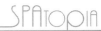

TREATMENTS

You think you know New Age? You don't know from New Age until you've had a *reiki* master–trained chakra therapist grab your coccyx bone so that she might sense vibrations that could lead to your aura being bathed in red light.

The seven chakras align with the spine, starting at the base, or root chakra, and working up to the crown. Each has an associated colour, emotion and spiritual aspect. Using intuition and touch by sensing subtle chakra vibrations, a therapist deciphers which of your chakras need to be balanced and what issues should be addressed.

You can talk about what's bothering you as you receive an incredible lymph drainage and Swedish massage while being hit with the prescribed multi-coloured lights. It's a massage *cum* psychology session *cum* spa disco.

A tripod light has coloured filters that are changed during the hour-long treatment. When the aura is bathed with certain colours it is meant to help one achieve balance. For example, if your root chakra is out of whack, stability in your finances could suffer. The solution? Bathe the root chakra in red. If your heart chakra is out of balance, it gets the green light. Certain colours are meant to energize, others to soothe.

It's a journey of self-discovery, and it's there for you when you're ready for it. But in case you're not, a purifying facial, featuring products from the Dr. Hauschka organic line, never hurt anyone. And not to worry — if you're coming in for a paraffin pedicure, the staff won't try to trick you into getting a chakra balance instead.

SERVICE

The well-trained staff members deftly explain the Chakra philosophy (and there's a lot to explain), welcome questions and clearly love what they do. If they were any more accommodating, they would be tripping over themselves.

BOTTOM LINE

Does having your aura bathed in brightly coloured lights actually do something? Who's to say? The end result is that you leave the spa feeling a lot more relaxed than when you arrived. And if you end up painting your bedroom red and purple, so much the better.

INFORMATION

Chakra Spa. 1184 Eglinton Avenue West, Toronto, ON. Phone: (416) 784-3438. E-mail: thechakraspa@bellnet.ca. The Chakra Colour Balancer is an hour long and costs CDN$70. The Chakra Purifier is 35 minutes and costs $65.

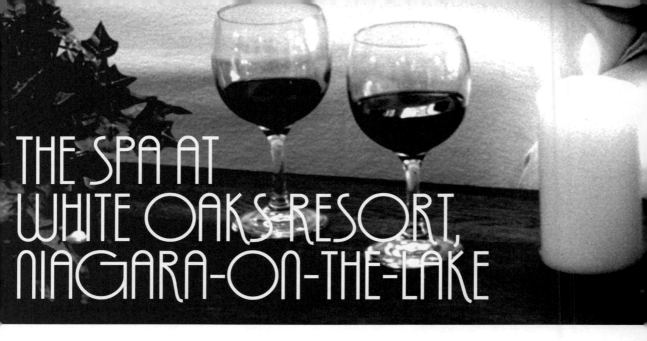

THE SPA AT WHITE OAKS RESORT, NIAGARA-ON-THE-LAKE

The Niagara Peninsula is the fertile heart of Ontario's wine-growing belt. And even though Niagara-on-the-Lake might seem like a quaint little refuge from the Big Smoke, there's more to this postcard town than homemade fudge. Growing and flourishing along with the local wineries that surround it, White Oaks Resort's spa now offers vinotherapy treatments that make good use of the region's indigenous offerings.

LOCATION

White Oaks is right off the Queen Elizabeth Way, about an hour and a half west of Toronto, which means there is no need for lengthy, ambling drives through Niagara's wine country. On the down side, that means no lengthy, ambling drives through Niagara's bucolic wine country. Even so, you're just minutes away from the Shaw Festival theatres, the Butterfly Conservatory, Casino Niagara, the Welland Canal, Niagara Falls, the Royal Niagara Golf Club, and a bunch of amazing wineries including Peller Estates, Inniskillin and Jackson-Triggs.

DESIGN

The brown-brick exterior hearkens back to Mike Brady's 1970s mien, while the garish gold panelling under the exterior windows makes for a facade only a mother could love. Once inside, though, it's a different world. Best to book rooms in the new tower, where the flavour is pure boutique-hotel chic: a palate of whites, beige, light wood and loads of sunshine. The expansive renovated spa has twenty-two treatment rooms decked out in a romantic faux-Tuscan finish, with burnished silver accents, earth-tone carpeting and fragrant air.

CLIENTELE

White Oaks is a convention centre, so on any given day you'll find Clarins con-ventioneers in one boardroom, and Fortinos in another. Bell may be utilizing the 140-seat amphitheatre, while the Investors Group have a team-building round-robin on the eight tennis courts. Incentive gifts have become big business, and convention-goers take full advantage via spa and golf bonuses.

TREATMENTS

The spa offers the usual aromatherapy facials, detoxifying seaweed wraps, manicures and pedicures, but it's their new vinotherapy treatments, like the "Nectar of Niagara," that set this one apart. It starts out with a fine scrub made from clay and grape pulp mixed together with some vino for good measure. After this, jugs of warm honey and wine are poured over the exfoliated body and massaged about, vaguely à la Mickey Rourke and Kim Basinger in *9½ Weeks*. Then comes a cocoon of thick towels whilst the mead-like body wrap sets. The grape byproducts are high in potent antioxidants called oligomeric proanthocyanidins, while the honey contains amino acids and vitamin B, providing hydration and nourishment to the skin.

Back on the massage table, the face is treated to a moisturizing facial of milk and honey, and then the chrysalis emerges from her terry-cloth cocoon and is helped into a hydrotherapy tub fuelled by milk and essential oils. A finishing rub of wine lotion and grapeseed oil completes this smorgasbord for the skin and the senses.

FOOD & DRINK

Lunch at White Oaks' restaurant, Liv, is an elegant affair. A glass of Hillebrand Dry Riesling is certainly in order — this being wine country, after all. The menu is full of old favourites with a gourmet twist; the BLT, for instance, features sugar-cured bacon, sliced avocado, Montasio cheese, tomatoes and watercress sprouts on a thick-sliced multigrain baguette, sided by sweet-potato chips. There's a good choice of sandwiches, salads, fish dishes and meatier meals and even pizza, albeit the stone-ground-wheat-and-hemp-flour variety. Dessert can be plucked from a sinful list — or better still, pick up a fresh fruit pie at a roadside stand on the drive home.

SERVICE

The staff is knowledgeable and friendly, bordering on overeager.

BOTTOM LINE

A vinotherapy and an afternoon spent trolling the wineries of Niagara will leave you feeling like a nouveau Beaujolais.

INFORMATION

The Spa at White Oaks Resort. 253 Taylor Road, Niagara-on-the-Lake, ON. Phone: 1-800-263-5766. Web: http://www.whiteoaksresort.com.

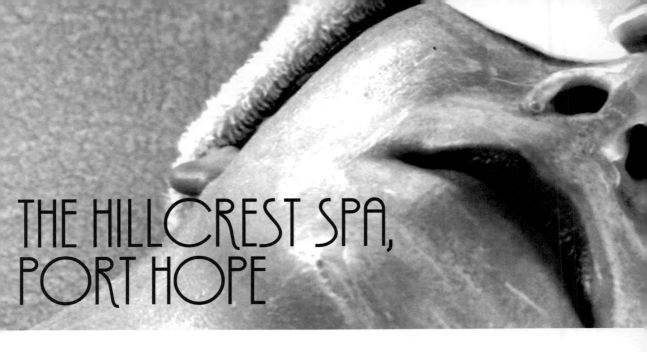

THE HILLCREST SPA, PORT HOPE

Oh, what a day it's been. What a week. What a life. Your computer is crashing, your best-looking fingernail has been bent in an excruciatingly painful direction, all you have in the fridge is a box of freezer-burned Lean Pockets and there's a naked photo of you in a compromising position making the rounds on the Internet. If any or all of these scenarios reflects your present lot, it's time to hightail it out of town to regroup and recover, and the Hillcrest Spa could be the answer to your R&R desires. A sister spa to the older Ste. Anne's in nearby Grafton, both are part of the Haldimand Hills Spa Village, a spa network that's just an hour out of Toronto.

LOCATION

Head east along Highway 401 for about 55 minutes, then turn off to be met by the sudden greenness of Haldimand Hills. A few curves and stops later, you'll pull into the Hillcrest Spa, a glorious Victorian mansion presiding over six forested hectares. It might just be the flora and fauna talking, but the same Lake Ontario that looks somewhat foreboding in Toronto becomes oddly romantic-looking here. You're also within walking distance of the historic town of Port Hope, home to Ontario's best-preserved Main Street.

DESIGN

Picture hardwood floors with fading runners strewn about, a baby grand piano, high ceilings, Irish antiques, Victorian chaises and crackling fireplaces. Comfy rooms with oversized beds could benefit from a professional decorator's touch, but are fortified with Aveda bath products and are bright and spacious. Outside, a plantation-style porch, sunburst foliage, blue skies and a sparkly lake make for genteel Canadiana.

CLIENTELE

Husbands and wives on anniversary retreats, a group of girlfriends from the States who say "y'all" a lot. A woman in a terry-cloth robe, alone, eating and reading a book, glowing.

TREATMENTS

The regular roundup of high-end services and quite a few interesting newbies. The Traditional Thai Massage incorporates aspects of reflexology, acupressure, shiatsu and yoga to stimulate energy lines, helping the body's inherent flow. You wear loose-fitting clothing and enter the dimly lit room — all beech hardwood, stonework walls and a big thick mat for getting down to business. You'll soon learn that there's little difference between what goes on here and what transpires in a WWE ring. Ryan the Thai masseur describes the course of this treatment — and then he is upon you.

With his powerful hands he stretches, pokes, twists, prods, karate chops and massages you. His expert technique brings you to the point of crying "Uncle!", but just before the brink you're brought back to cooing "Oh, baby." This one is not for the timid.

The Moor Wrap Hydromassage is also a little on the wild side. Penny, who has all of the Aveda products and accoutrements laid out on a gurney-style massage table, asks you to smell different bottles so as to choose the essences to be added to various muds and creams.

And so it begins. First, lying naked on the massage table (with a towel tastefully covering your nether regions), you undergo a medium-strength dry brushing to remove dead skin and baked-on grime (you get to keep the cool brush). A quick shower, then a coating of the dark brown mud that doubles as a detoxifying body stocking. You're cocooned for twenty minutes while you receive deep scalp and foot massages, then it's time to hop into the hydro tub, which has been fortified with more mud kicked with pine essence. Penny leaves the room for a moment and re-emerges wearing a bathing suit to hose you down.

Next up, the Vichy rain shower. You tread lightly along the slippery tiled floor, hop back onto the massage table and are rolled under the six massaging, soothing shower heads. Then it's time to dry the table, dry yourself and lie down for a thick application of moisturizing lotion.

FOOD & DRINK

Since the Hillcrest's capacity maxes out at sixteen guests, the kitchen can accommodate all dining needs; in any case, the printed menus are full of choice and are changed daily. Breakfast entails all the good stuff, including hotcakes, sausages, yogurt and granola. Even so, some overnighters can't bear to bring themselves to the table: "I was lying in this huge four-poster bed thinking, 'I can go downstairs for bacon and eggs, or I can stay in bed for another half-hour.' I decided I can get eggs and bacon in Toronto anytime," said one woman to her friend, who nodded in agreement.

The food is fresh and plentiful, if somewhat ordinary. Lunch could be potato-leek soup, grilled-chicken and spinach salad, tuna wraps and herb-punched tea biscuits straight from the oven. Dinners have more lofty ambitions: seared scallop and shrimp napped with raspberry vinaigrette, walnut-and-cranberry-stuffed chicken breast, chocolate hazelnut pâté. Best is tea (fresh-baked cookies, cream-cheese-and-cuke sandwiches, fruit, assorted hot beverages) laid out at 2 p.m., just as you're getting hit by those post–Thai massage hunger pangs.

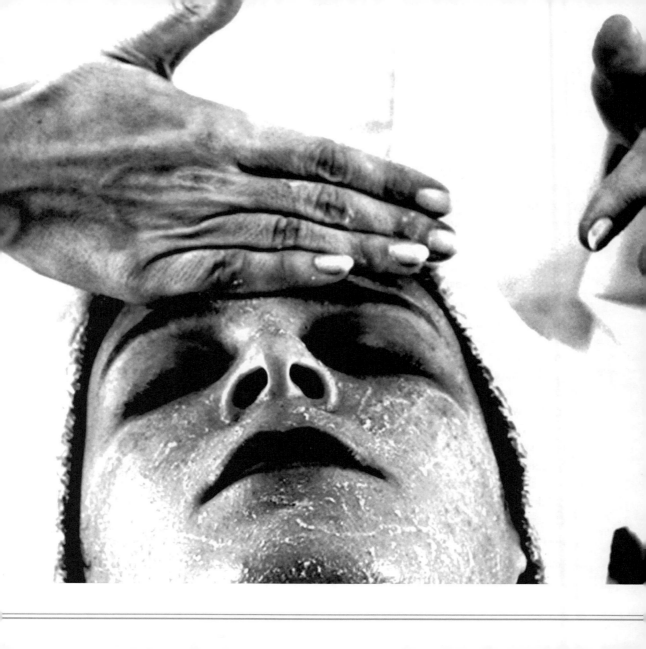

SERVICE

The staff is as chipper as the morning songbirds, especially Margarete the innkeeper, who prances around, grasping guests' hands, doling out local history lessons and reuniting wandering spa partners amid this Fawlty Towers–esque setup.

BOTTOM LINE

The Hillcrest is not a day spa. You come here for at least a night, but more often two. Meals are a terry-cloth-robe affair, and you book whatever treatments suit your fancy. If you're looking for some solace and good-natured pampering, think about heading for these hills.

INFORMATION

The Hillcrest Spa. 175 Dorset Street West, Port Hope, ON. Phone: 1-888-346-6772. Web: http://www.haldimandhills.com.
Moor Wrap Hydromassage is an hour and a half long and costs CDN$125. Thai Massage lasts an hour and costs $85. Overnight packages at the Hillcrest start at $245 for the Last-Minute Spa Break, to the Five-Night Total Transformation starting at $1,125 a person. All packages include accommodations, meals, tea time, and varying degrees of spa allowances.

HALDIMAND HILLS SPA VILLAGE, GRAFTON

Luxury spa vacations are everything from the perfect antidote for the midwinter blues to a quick summer getaway. Where else can you work off your cake and eat it, too? That said, on the one-hour train ride east from Toronto, I felt mildly anxious about my five-day spa trip. What if I have to starve to achieve my five-pound weight-loss goal? (Or, worse, what if the food's no good?) What if they laugh at my lacklustre fitness level? What if I'm bored, or — and this is a real possibility — die from e-mail withdrawal?

I needn't have worried. As I pull into the front drive of Ste. Anne's Spa, it's love at first sight. I can immediately tell that Haldimand Hills Spa Village is about gain without pain.

LOCATION

The sprawling wellness complex was born in 1981, when owner Jim Corcoran bought a charming 1858 fieldstone château and began creating a laid-back spa retreat. All stone walls and well-heeled turrets and gables, surrounded by more than 200 hectares of woods, farmland and gardens, the village is centred around Ste. Anne's Country Inn & Spa in Grafton, where I'll be spending my spa holiday. Nearby is the Hillcrest Victorian Inn & Spa in Port Hope. And just down the road from Ste. Anne's is Maison Santé, a fitness centre where I'll be spending a lot of time getting daily doses of personal training and taking group classes. There are also various multi-roomed cottages dotted amidst the property for team-building retreats or gaggles of pals who want extra privacy. Nature hikes are a must, and Lake Ontario is just o'er yonder.

DESIGN

Ste. Anne's is like a grown-up playground featuring fitness classes, outdoor activities and Aveda products. The mood is that of a relaxed country estate with crackling fireplaces, oversized couches, bedrooms painted in cheery colours and containing four-poster beds that require either a footstool or a running leap to mount. The dining room overlooks the glorious English gardens, where there are cabanas (for alfresco massages), chaises longues, hammocks, a lovely pool, an outdoor fieldstone grotto hot tub and mineral baths, tennis courts and walking paths. There are about two dozen spa rooms, plus the expansive relaxation room one floor down.

CLIENTELE

Men and women in thick white terry-cloth robes are splayed across handsome couches and the outdoor lounges, drunk on peppermint stone wraps and De-stress with Breath lessons. It's like a grown-up slumber party at a rich relative's summer estate. At the pool, which is open from dawn to dusk, I take in the last bit of daylight before dinner. While I read my book, I can't help but eavesdrop on two forty-something women draped over flotation noodles. One says, "Look at that sky. Look at those puffy clouds. And that tree…" "Here comes Rose," says the other. Rose approaches, yawning. "I was lying in a hammock," she says. A man swims laps while his wife practises yoga near the shallow end.

Life is good.

And the buzz around the spa is great. Even the men are talking about their very first facials and shiatsu massages like giddy schoolgirls. I overhear four friends talking over lunch in the dining room. "What did you do yesterday?" one pair asks the other. "We were exfoliating," they laugh. "And today, we're moulting." Everyone laughs together.

TREATMENTS

My first circuit-training session goes well. Then I have a ninety-minute personal yoga lesson, followed by a Thai massage (which is like having yoga done to you). I go for a little nature walk, then take a meditation and stretch class to get in touch with my "true authentic self." (I'm using spa-speak; this is good.) The meditation is so calming — all pillows and soft, guiding voices — that we lose a few to sleep along the way.

One of the most talked-about treatments at Ste. Anne's is the moor mud bath, a house specialty. "Other than us, the nearest ones are in California," explains my spa technician, Brenda. The mineral-rich mud is composed of Leda clay, a "rock flour" eroded off of the Canadian Shield and carried away via glacial meltwater, then deposited as sediment on the bottom of the prehistoric Champlain Sea (a body of water that once covered the Ottawa Valley and St. Lawrence Lowlands, including the current sites of Ottawa and Montreal).

The treatment starts with ten minutes in a thick cloud of eucalyptus steam "to raise the body temperature and open the pores, so they can better accept the properties of the mud," says Brenda. Then you rinse off and shimmy into a tub of mud. It feels amazing, like thick chocolate pudding. After fifteen minutes of penetrating warmth and healing earth, you rinse off and lie down under an eight-headed Vichy shower that soothes the back and kneads the flesh. My eyelids feel like leaden manhole covers.

SERVICE

My first appointment is a fitness assessment with Jared Lloyd, a good-natured, square-jawed personal trainer and bodybuilder. He spends an hour taking readings of my height, weight, blood pressure and heart rate. First, he uses calipers to measure fat in key areas (thankfully, the butt isn't one of them), putting me through push-ups, sit-ups, jumps and a cardio test. Firm but fair. Over the following days I will spend much quality time with Jared during private cardio and weight-training workouts as well as group classes. You'd be hard pressed to meet a more professional and likable fellow. From Brenda at the mud baths to Shawna in the reflexology room to the cleaning crew and wait staff, everyone treats me with the warmth and hospitality befitting a country home.

SPATOPIA

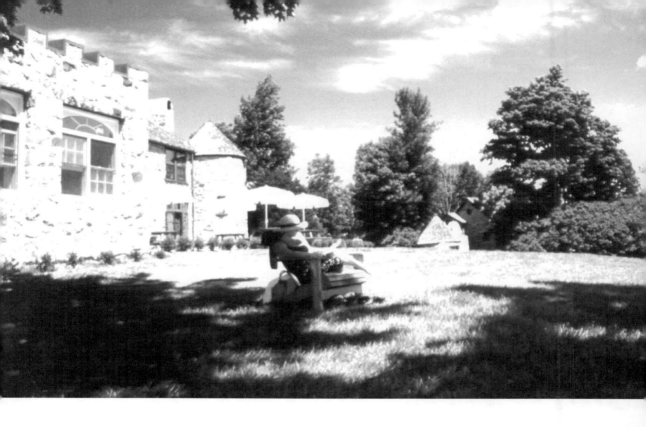

HALDIMAND HILLS SPA VILLAGE

This network of striking buildings is perfect for exercise, mud wraps, afternoon tea and everything in between. The Five-Night Total Transformation package includes accommodations and meals, a CDN$200 spa allowance and unlimited group class-es; a fitness assessment and personal training sessions are options.

FOOD & DRINK

Fuel up at breakfast with hearty asparagus-and-cheese omelettes, whole-wheat toast, fresh fruit and a couple of cups of strong coffee; or, fresh-baked pastries, waffles and a morning special, like blueberry pancakes. No alcohol is sold here, but guests take full advantage of the spa's BYOB policy to accompany dinners like steak with borde-laise sauce, lunches of Caesar salad with seared tuna, and desserts that include the likes of peach cobbler and chocolate pâté. But best is the 3 p.m. standing appointment: tea time. Oh, Jared's great and all, but he can't compete with mini sour cherry scones with thick Devon cream and preserves, or the crisp flaxseed cookies still warm from the oven... Isn't this kind of like eating chocolates while jogging? Beside me, two young women finish taking tea on the veranda. "Hel-*looo?*" says the taller one, dabbing her mouth with a linen napkin. "I'm at a spa, and I'm eating cheese and brownies!" Sounds decadent, and some of the choices are just that, but the food is all about fresh, flavourful, perfectly portioned gourmet spa cuisine.

BOTTOM LINE

After five days of extreme spa-ing consisting of hours of treatments and days of fresh air and fruitful exercise, simply put, you won't know what hit you.

INFORMATION

Haldimand Hills Spa Village, near Grafton, ON. Phone: 1-888-346-6772.
Web: http://www.haldimandhills.com.

SPATOPIA

LE SPA, HOTEL LE ST-JAMES, MONTREAL

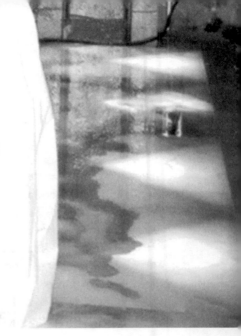

t was just over a decade ago — late-night TV host Arsenio Hall was at the height of his popularity, McDonald's had just introduced pizza to its menu and in Montreal the separatists' calls for change were building. The once-lively St. Catherine Street had begun to resemble a ghost town, and as for Old Montreal — well, no one but tourists ever went there.

It's amazing what a little time can do for a city. Within the past few years, no fewer than seven boutique hotels have popped up in this historic part of town, and with the opening of Le St-James, the stakes got that much higher. Staying at this über-decadent hotel is like event slumbering, and booking an appointment at its personal spa turns the event into a downright extravaganza.

LOCATION

Le St-James is just a stone's throw from the banks of the St. Lawrence River and the birthplace of Montreal. Hop aboard a kitschy-fun calèche for a whirlwind tour of this architecturally gifted area, which is especially romantic by night. Clip-clopping down narrow cobblestone streets that have seen more than 350 years of history feels like a trip back in time. Among other attractions, you'll see the Old Sulpician Seminary (the oldest building in the city), Place Jacques-Cartier, the Old Port, City Hall and Nôtre-Dame Basilica. The area is also loaded with museums and galleries, trendy shops and fine French eats.

DESIGN

The spa is so highly designed it could double as a set in a James Bond movie. The entrance into the sole treatment room is a curved steel wall that locks electronically. Once inside, though, it's strictly Old World (save for the gorgeous under-lit onyx floor, Denon stereo and Vichy shower). This basement area is the former gunpowder room of the old merchant bank that the hotel was built on, with original brick ceilings, archways and stone walls from the centuries-old rampart. Today, with melting candles jutting out from nooks in the walls, it's all very soothing.

    The rooms and suites in the St-James are every bit as artful and full of surprises. Montreal interior designer Jacques Bouchard amassed a collection of antiques, French tapestries, European inlays, fine art and woven rugs, and somehow made it all work. Every room is different and equally beautiful, from the two-storey ceilings and original hardwood floors of the heritage suites to the decadent Italian marble bathrooms in every room. This is one boutique hotel where opulence reigns and minimalism is for suckers.

CLIENTELE

CEOs and celebrities who covet class and privacy.

TREATMENTS

Imagine having a spa to yourself. That's basically the deal here. Hélène rules the roost, and offers a good range of massages (Swedish, sports, deep tissue, stone, Vichy shower or kinetic), exfoliation treatments, body wraps and peels. She's a talented masseuse and will do your body good, but the best part is still to come. She gives you a key and says, "The change room is all yours." The hyperbolic steel entrance slides open, you pad down the hall and enter another gorgeous room of archways, marble, frosted glass, fluffy towels, Fuji water and four doors. The first one is a toilet — not too exciting. The second is a sauna, large enough to hold fifteen. The third is a steam room, large enough for eight and already steamed up, and then there's the shower. This engineering feat has regular, rainshower, hand-held and four-side shower heads. Ostensibly you're meant to use only one head at a time, but try them all at once for extreme showering. The men's room has duplicate amenities, but the design is a little more masculine, with greys, slate and metallics instead of wood and marble. About half the patrons of the spa are men.

FOOD & DRINK

Since the hotel is surrounded by five-star restaurants and hipster hangouts such as Cube and Soto, the property has wisely turned its focus to room service, even though breakfast, afternoon tea and bar snacks may be taken in the magnificent two-tiered dining room on the entrance level. So, what does room service mean at the St-James? A $12 cup of joe, for starters. The full-service kitchen also offers gourmet treats, including Beluga caviar (50 grams) with blinis and cream for $300, or the chef's $21 cheeseburger. There are also late-night snacks, including vegetarian pizza ($20) and chicken wings ($25 for 12). Sure, it's over the top, but imagine eating crème brûlée while luxuriating in a down-swathed antique bed.

SERVICE

The hotel has earned the Leading Small Hotels of the World insignia, making it part of an international network of five-star hotels that meet the highest standards of excellence and quality in all aspects of service. And so it is that every need at the St-James is seen to posthaste with efficiency and grace. This includes a daily in-room weather report card, a touch-screen phone system you'll need an engineering degree to operate, Penhaligon's toiletries from England and bedtime truffles. There's even a free shoe-shining service; simply fill out the form, pop your shoes in the special bag and put them out for pickup before 1 a.m. By 6 a.m., they'll be calling you Twinkle Toes.

BOTTOM LINE

If you're not duly impressed by the sumptuousness, service and pedigree of the St-James, then there's just no pleasing you.

INFORMATION

Hotel Le St-James. 355 Rue Saint-Jacques, Montreal, QC. Phone: (514) 841-3111 or 1-866-841-3111. Web: http://www.hotellestjames.com. There are 61 rooms, including 38 suites. Pricing is based on square footage and ranges from about CDN$400 to $5,000 a night (for the penthouse suite). An hour-long Swedish massage costs $95 and includes use of the private sauna, steam room and that kicking shower.

OVARIUM FLOATATION BATHS, MONTREAL

n the 1980 sci-fi thriller *Altered States*, a Harvard research scientist uses a sensory deprivation tank and hallucinogenic drugs to find the fundamental truth behind various states of consciousness. But it's not long before his mind-altering experiments go awry and he pays... the ultimate price. So, as I found myself easing into a coffin-like floatation bath filled with super-saturated salt water at Montreal's Ovarium, let's just say I had some misgivings. Grave misgivings....

LOCATION

The copper-topped former bank building flanks a busy street corner in the residential Petite Patrie district, near Montreal's vibrant Little Italy.

DESIGN

The first thing you notice upon entering the vast space is the overwhelming smell of chlorine. And looking around at the coat check racks near the front and people shuffling about in sandals, you get the feeling you might be in a glorified bathhouse. But some nice touches negate any seedy notions. There are soaring ceilings, walls of pale yellow and white, marble floors, comfy chairs, gurgling water features and some ferns and fans. Stacks of sound systems by the reception area pipe optional meditation tracks into each of the six floatation baths, and there is also a handful of massage therapy rooms.

Although it may sound intimidating, it's a quietly businesslike, non-threatening environment. There are two lounge areas, one at the front reception area for pre-treatment, the other towards the back where you relax, post-float. The latter is outfitted in teak loungers and features a fish tank, and is so deathly quiet that one almost feels compelled to hold mirrors under people's noses.

CLIENTELE

There are loads of regulars streaming through, and men and women (ranging in age from their twenties to fifties) are in equal proportions. On a Thursday afternoon, the place was at maximum capacity, full of city-dwellers going back to the womb for an hour or two and getting regular massages via multi-pack memberships.

SPATOPIA

TREATMENTS

The point of floating naked in a tank is to be in a weightless environment and experience sensory deprivation. Here's how the glossy brochure explains it: "Comfortably stretched out in your personal egg-shaped bath, you will gently move towards a profound state of well-being and relaxation, towards a feeling of infinity… Floating in a weightless environment frees up to 90 percent of the potential of our central nervous system's energy. The resulting biochemical balancing produces numerous long-term effects, including profound relaxation, harmonization of the two hemispheres of the brain, normalization of sleep patterns, stabilization of emotions and dependencies, enhanced powers of concentration and creativity." Sounds sublimely New Agey. Let's give her a spin.

To start with, you remain completely buoyant because the tank contains a solution of body-temperature H_2O containing 2,000 cups of Epsom salts (akin to the Dead Sea). Besides the salt, the water is chlorine-treated and bacteria-free, and fresh air is piped into the tank. You can leave the internal blue light on or off (they suggest off), and there's a handy call button should you reach a state of consciousness you're not quite able to deal with. You also have the choice of leaving the door of your bath open, partially open or closed (it's on a counterweight system). There are private showers in each room, with towels, soap, shampoo, conditioner and cotton swabs. They're very adamant about you cleaning your ears properly afterwards (because of the salt, perhaps?). Hair dryers and hair care products are also provided in a separate area.

Step into your private room (all of which have appropriate names, such as Neptune), undress, shower, ease into the tank and shut the door. Off goes the light; on comes the mood music. The brain flickers. It takes a few minutes to relax and get acclimatized. For instance, I felt a bit of a chill and worried that the chlorine would ruin my new dye job. But you quickly ease into the peace and quiet, and fifty minutes ends up feeling like five. You know your hour is over when you hear a chorus of angels singing. Literally. Rest assured, they're coming from the sound system; it's not just in your head.

Ovarium also offers an impressive roster of massage techniques to treat everything from backaches to stress. Options include Amma, Californian, Lymphatic Drainage, Esalen, Jin Shin Do, Shiatsu, Sports, Swedish and Trager.

SERVICE

The young staffers, decked out in designer eyewear, give this New Age concept a decidedly modern vibe. If you're a first-timer, one of them will happily give you the grand tour and describe in meticulous detail everything that will happen before, during and after your float. They'll also bring you tea to drink in the relaxation area while you zone back in.

BOTTOM LINE

Floating around in a deep, dark tank filled with salt water may not be everyone's cup of tea, but I found it to be a Calgon moment — taken to the extreme. No sight, no sound, no gravity. Just you.

INFORMATION

Ovarium. 400 Rue Beaubien East (corner of Rue St. Denis), QC. Montreal. Metro Station: Beaubien. Phone: (514) 271-7515 or 1-877-FLOTTER. Web: http://www.ovarium.com. An hour in the tank costs CDN$42, or $107 for a three-session membership. Hour-long massages cost $56, or $154 for a three-session membership.

SPATOPIA

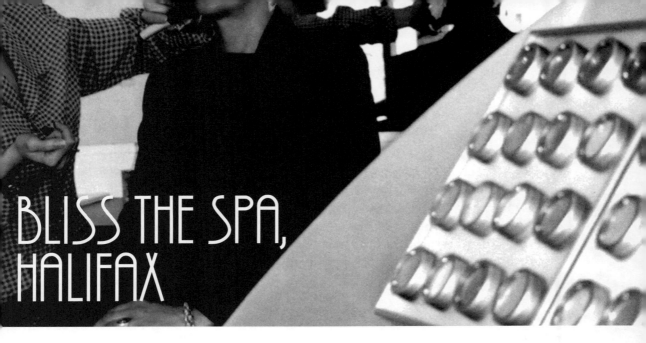

BLISS THE SPA, HALIFAX

Farewell to Halifax, sleepy seaside town of yore, and hello to a newly pumped-up city going through a redevelopment renaissance. There's still room for the prideful bagpipers who play for the ice-cream-licking hordes on the harbourfront boardwalk, but change is afoot. It is a red sky this night (to use seafaring parlance), owing in part to oil exploration and the cruise liners now docking in port. Down home is turning upscale, with expensive restaurants, trendy shops and the new Bliss the Spa overlooking Halifax Harbour. Could it be that a sailor's delight will soon consist of thoughts of a gentleman's facial and ear candling?

Photo by Amy Rosen

LOCATION

Bishop's Landing, a newly sprung waterfront complex near Halifax's south end, is home to 204 yuppie-approved apartments; Bliss, the 1,100-square-metre day spa; and Bish World Cuisine (a restaurant serving neighbourhood-inspired cuisine such as Nova Scotia smoked salmon on blinis with crème fraiche).

Just beyond the Landing is a compact city built for strolling. Across the street is Alexander Keith's Nova Scotia Brewery Tour, a lively and thirst-quenching history lesson at the Brewery Market. In the same historic building is the Saturday farmer's market, where visitors can work their way through a labyrinth of colourful stalls while picking up everything from bunches of organic carrots to fresh-cut flowers and free-range chickens.

Minutes away is Point Pleasant Park, full of woodsy trails and home in the summer to theatre with Shakespeare by the Sea. Also nearby is the Pier 21 museum, the Maritime Museum of the Atlantic and the Art Gallery of Nova Scotia.

DESIGN

The ten treatment rooms, hair salon, pedicure lounge and café are done in hues of brandy cream and bluegrass, with pale hardwood floors and complementary tile work. The showstoppers are the floor-to-ceiling windows at the entrance that welcome the sunshine and harbour views. The well-equipped fitness centre is open to all, and a climb up its spiral staircase leads to the spa's rooftop hot tub and pool.

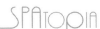

SPATOPIA

CLIENTELE

The first to discover Bliss were the Haligonians who reside at Bishop's Landing. Then it was cruise ship passengers in need of detoxification after one too many midnight buffets. And, as always, confused gents come to buy gift certificates on the sly for their wives. But no sailors as of yet.

TREATMENTS

Inspired by its surroundings, Bliss offers a goodly supply of water-based treatments, including a Revitalizing Marine Wrap that utilizes special mud to firm drooping flesh. The wrap begins with Italian Comfort Zone brand exfoliation gel, which rubs off like eraser bits. Then comes the green marine-sediment mud, which has a firming effect on the skin and is said to speed regeneration from within deep tissue. Once in full Incredible Hulk mode, you're wrapped in plastic and swathed in towels and a thick comforter for twenty minutes. At this point, some people experience a hot sensation on the skin while others feel a dry cold breeze as the fucus (brown marine algae) goes to work, aided by naturally occurring chlorine, potassium, calcium, magnesium, iron and iodine. End result: increased elasticity and smooth, soft skin.

The Refining Algae Facial involves about a dozen steps, including a prep tonic, exfoliation, a neutralizing tonic, a massage, a mask of calming alginate that dries like rubber, and an expert makeup application at the end. That last part may lead to some head scratching amongst regular spa-goers, as makeup is usually verboten after a facial (it clogs the pores of newly buffed skin). Not here. Bliss uses the Jane Iredale line of micronized mineral makeup, which is non-comedogenic (does not contribute to acne), oil-free, anti-inflammatory, and has SPF factors between 17 and 20.

SERVICE

A young, can-do team of Halifax men and women welcomes questions and conversation. Ask for Dawn, a pixie-haired dead ringer for Anne of Green Gables.

BOTTOM LINE

Bliss is in the right place at the right time, and has of-the-moment treatments being dispensed by a knowledgeable staff. Looks like smooth sailing on the horizon.

INFORMATION

Bliss the Spa. Bishop's Landing (1477 Lower Water Street), Halifax, NS.
Phone: (902) 420-8555. Web: http://www.blissthespa.com.
The Revitalizing Marine Wrap and Algae Refining Facial are each CDN$95. Bliss also has a full line of body polishes and wraps, facials, massages and nail and salon treatments.

SPIRIT SPA, HALIFAX

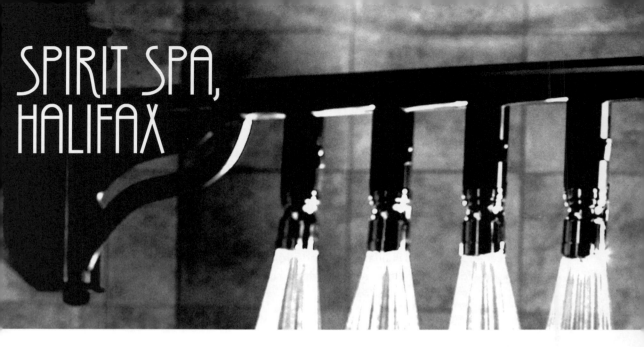

The organic products used at the new Spirit Spa in Halifax are not all about 1970s egg yolk shampoo rinsed with Gee Your Hair Smells Terrific conditioner. These are high-end, handmade, all-natural goodies dished out in downtown digs where the vibe is anything but a leftover from the Age of Aquarius. Which isn't to say it's not about healing, peace and tranquility, because it's all of those, too.

Spirit is also about squeezing a Nooner massage into a hectic workweek, or taking the afternoon off to revel in a marine-based urban spa package. This downtown spa is here to aid the work-weary urban professional in the art of organic relaxation, especially during those moments when the moon might be in the seventh house, but the courier didn't deliver those contracts on time.

LOCATION

The 100-year-old Barrington Street building that houses the spa faced the wrecking ball when Haligonian spa owner Linda Brigley and her partners decided to restore it to its former glory. "Our business is about rejuvenation and renewal, and we wanted to do some urban renewal project as part of our development," she says.

It was a good fit. Barrington Street itself is currently undergoing a slow but sure revitalization, whereby seedy greasy spoons and boarded-up blocks are being gentrified and turned into shops and restaurants, such as the UpCountry home décor store next door and chic Chives Canadian Bistro across the street.

DESIGN

The soaring third-storey space is done up in a colour palate of soft lime-Popsicle green, basil and grey. The original rough-hewn beams, posts and light maple panels are used wherever possible, while sunlight beams into the large, atrium-like relaxation room. From the reception area to the four treatment rooms and Vichy wet room, the look is simple, clean and gender-neutral. It's got contemporary flair with a Zen-inspired left hook.

CLIENTELE

Consider Spirit an urban spa — its clientele consists largely of downtown professionals, with almost an equal split between men and women. Brigley, who worked in business management in Halifax herself before opening the spa, says her clients are much like her: "It's about relaxing the way they want to." Those wanting to get in and get out in the middle of the day come for the express pedicures, with two aestheticians working at once. But most come to dive in and check out of the rat race, if only for their lunch hour.

TREATMENTS

Specialty treatments, all with clever names, include packages like Day at the Beach, which features a sea scrub, a sunless tan application, foil highlights, a haircut and a pedicure. It almost sounds better than actually going to the beach. The Mani-Pedi Club is also a bright idea, akin to a coffee-club card — if you buy five services, you get one free.

It was hard to pass on the Urban Rainforest body treatment. A head-to-toe exfoliant using marine-based products from France that slough away stress (and a cell or two of dead skin) is followed by a seven-headed Vichy shower that massages you down to your core. After the shower, a remineralizing gel mask, including lavender, basil, ylang-ylang and other sea-based ingredients, wraps you in a twenty-minute aromatherapy straitjacket, and you receive a calming scalp massage while the mask penetrates. You're polished off with another rinse, Vichy-style, followed by a hydrating body moisturizing lotion.

The Sweet Skin Facial, meant to firm and revitalize, uses a handmade organic skin care line called Eminence. These Hungarian products are all based on fruits, herbs and vegetables, with the facials being custom blended for your skin type. You get your own prescription at the end, which includes a skin diagnosis — such as combo/oily and dehydration — plus, of course, the listing of products and treatments you might want to buy. The facial starts with a rosehip and maize exfoliant that helps the other products work to their full potential by preparing the skin. A stimulating lime mask kicked up with hot paprika is professionally administered and makes the skin feel extremely hot (to the point where you might think something very bad is happening), but cools down as soon as it's removed. It gets results on a par with a doctor-administered acid peel. But, of course, this one's all-natural.

Best was the sour-cherry masque made from cherry pulp, honey, lemon juice, cinnamon and bioflavonoids. Spritzes of rosehip tonic — which is good for oily skin, as it controls the sebaceous glands — were also welcome, as was the Couperose-C serum, an antioxidant and anti-irritant that's good for revving up microcirculation. The finishing Rosehip Whip Moisturizer is light and great for summer because it absorbs right into the skin. Then you leave, with your complexion all peaches and cream.

SERVICE

As you enter at ground level, the music piped into the building sets the tone. Fruity water and juices, herbal teas and decaf are there for the drinking. Catered lunches include healthy sandwiches and salads such as organic baby greens with salmon. As for treatments, book with Angela, who's perhaps the most informative and skilled aesthetician you'll meet. She's even got stories: on a recent morning, she awoke to find her seven-year-old daughter spreading organic sour-cherry facial product on her toast (the contents being organic, the fancy jar is stored in the fridge). "It wouldn't hurt her, because it's all-natural," Angela says. "But that was some very expensive jam."

BOTTOM LINE

From the Frette bathrobes and luxe organic products to the sunny, gender-neutral space and spot-on location, Spirit Spa is so well conceived and smart-looking you'd think it was a chain. And it should be. Only in Halifax, eh? Pity.

INFORMATION

Spirit Spa. 1566 Barrington Street, Halifax, NS Phone: (902) 431-8100;
Web: http://www.spiritspa.ca.
The Sweet Skin Facial lasts seventy-five minutes and costs CDN$75, while the ninety-minute Urban Rainforest Body Treatment is $120.

OTHER CANADIAN DESTINATION SPAS

THE HILLS HEALTH RANCH

In the hills of British Columbia's Cariboo Country (near 108 Mile Lake), settle in for a six-night Inches Off package in the lodge or the cozy chalets. Included are calorie-counted meals, juice elixirs, vitamins, a fitness assessment, lifestyle and nutrition advice, exercise classes, cross-country skiing — and a hayride! Phone: (250) 791-5225. Web: http://www.spabc.com.

MOUNTAIN TREK FITNESS RETREAT & HEALTH SPA

Located at Ainsworth Hot Springs near Nelson, B.C., Mountain Trek has a FitPlan Weight Loss retreat for those who are serious about shedding pounds. One- to three-week packages include a personal fitness appraisal and programs, daily yoga/stretch classes, guided hikes (or, in the winter, snowshoeing), guided weight workouts, massage, a nutrition consultation, gourmet meals and a spa cuisine cooking class. Phone: 1-800-661-5161. Web: http://www.mountaintrek.com.

SPA EASTMAN

An hour east of Montreal, where there's also a city location, the country's largest destination spa (forty-four rooms spread among seven pavilions) has Mount Orford as a backdrop. The Relaxation and Vitality packages (minimum three nights) include a naturopathic nutrition evaluation, a naturopath-supervised personalized cure program, lodging, meals, fitness activities, access to the pools and hammam, and spa treatments. Phone: 1-800-665-5272. Web: http://www.eastmanspa.com.

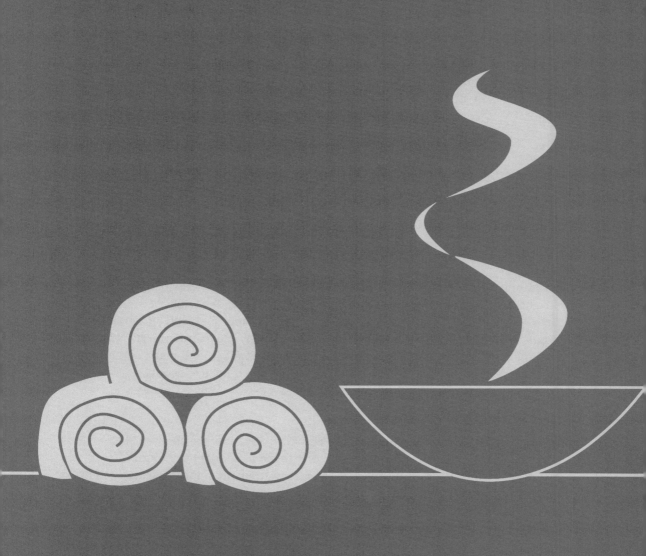

SPAS IN THE UNITED STATES

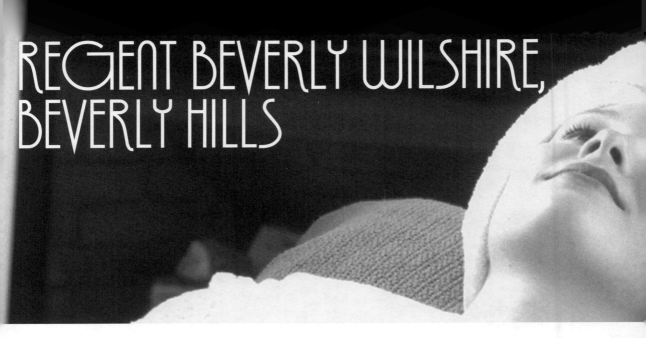

REGENT BEVERLY WILSHIRE, BEVERLY HILLS

The movie *Pretty Woman* may have won Julia Roberts the title of America's sweetheart, but at the same time it also cemented the Regent Beverly Wilshire's place as a hotel icon. More than just a backdrop for the popular hooker-turned-Cinderella flick, the hotel became a central character in itself — from its glorious European architecture and grand marble lobby entrances to its sudsy deep-dish tubs and the ever-helpful concierge. Not one to look a gift horse in the mouth, the hotel and spa have wisely pounced upon their film-induced fame by offering up deals such as the Pretty Woman Suite Getaway, and their signature six-hour head-to-toe spa package, appropriately called the Pretty Woman.

LOCATION

The hotel is situated at the famed Beverly Hills intersection of Rodeo Drive and Wilshire Boulevard, where the average store sells panties that cost more than the GDP of most developing nations. You know the drill: Gucci, Louis Vuitton, Saks Fifth Avenue and the like — just the sort of snobby places that wouldn't let poor Julia's character in during the movie.

Times have changed, though, and now some of these high-end shops have actually joined forces with the Beverly Wilshire for their Pretty Woman Suite getaways. "Starter gifts" and VIP store invites include a $1,000 gift certificate toward a Lana Marks signature alligator handbag, or a cultured pearl and a $1,250 gift certificate from Mikimoto, which you might use towards a Tahitian pearl necklace.

DESIGN

Grand marble and sweeping ceilings, frescoes, chandeliers, lush silks, wools and tassels, all done up in vibrant hues. The hotel's Dining Room, Lobby Lounge and The Bar (you've got to love it when they call a thing a thing) are all very handsome places where you can alternatively enjoy a formal meal, a full tea service or a high-ball next to the baby grand piano. The pool area has a comely Mediterranean vibe that screams Hollywood glam, but sadly the spa is a faded beauty in need of a face-lift — or at least a few strategically placed Botox injections.

The treatment rooms are spacious, homey and full of high-tech spa equipment. But brown shag carpet? Feh. The spa is located in an annexed part of the hotel, and oddly the check-in and change rooms are in different buildings (meaning you'll have to walk through the pool area in your robe). But even though the spa is small (just four treatment rooms), you've also got the fitness centre, hair salon, steam and sauna at your disposal.

CLIENTELE

Reformed Hollywood playboy Warren Beatty lived in the Veranda Suite for eleven years, but today the lobby is full of happy tourists snapping pictures. The Lobby Lounge is also a local hangout for wealthy octogenarians, as evidenced by the abundance of blue hair and bifocal-sporting shufflers named Sammy. The spa is frequented mainly by locals, as well as jet-lagged travellers.

"I have a client who was very depressed after her husband died," aesthetician Estella says. "She was seeing a psychiatrist for a year, but then started coming to me for three hours of spa treatments each month." Now the woman feels better, but more importantly, she looks fabulous.

TREATMENTS

There are a good assortment of packages on offer, from the Regent Royal and Traveler's Retreat, to the Men's Revitalizer and Wedding Day Bliss. The Pretty Woman spa package is the biggest blowout. It includes an hour-long personal training session, a choice of fifty-minute massage, a Rejuvenating Facial, a manicure, Perfect Pedicure (with paraffin), makeup application, hair wash and blow dry, and poolside lunch. It costs US$700 and does not include a date with Richard Gere. So really, why bother?

Instead, try the Pineapple Coconut Crunch Sugar Glow. Meant to bring dry skin back from the brink, the treatment uses pure cane sugar from Fiji, natural coconut oil rich in vitamins and antioxidants, and pineapple oil full of helpful alpha hydroxyl. It starts with a dry brushing to aid circulation (you try to ignore the cirrus cloud of skin flakes hovering above you), then the sugar mixture is massaged on, followed by a deep scrubbing with a loofah (you won't bleed, even though it feels like it) to remove more dead skin. This is wiped off with hot towels before a thick application of moisturizer is slathered on — it's advisable to take a steam and shower to let it all sink in. End result: smooth, youthful, moisturized skin.

SERVICE

Estella was a true pro, and service throughout the hotel was accommodating and kindly.

BOTTOM LINE

Having just celebrated its seventy-fifth birthday (although it's had work, so it looks maybe half that), this place is a ritzed-up ode to old-school Hollywood, which is pretty cool, actually. When you stay at the Beverly Wilshire, the hotel's Rolls-Royce will take you anywhere within three miles of the property. Imagine: all scrubbed, polished and done up at the spa, then whisked away in a luxury car. Just be sure you make it home before midnight.

INFORMATION

Regent Beverly Wilshire Spa. 9500 Wilshire Boulevard, Beverly Hills, CA. Phone: (310) 275-5200 or (310) 385-7023 (spa). Web: http://www.regenthotels.com/beverlywilshire. The Pineapple Coconut Crunch Sugar Glow lasts 50 minutes and costs US$130.

SPATOPIA

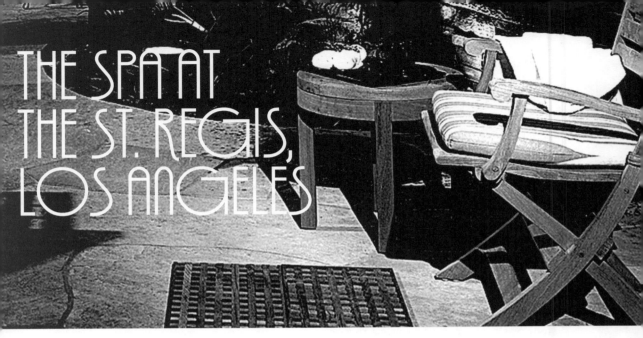

THE SPA AT THE ST. REGIS, LOS ANGELES

The asymmetrical bob, leg warmers and Valley Girl–speak were the hallmarks of the 1980s — an age of Smurfs, *Ghostbusters*, *Family Ties* and Bananarama. Although many of us remember it fondly as the John Hughes era, these were also the Reagan years. The Century Plaza Hotel was built in 1984, just before President Reagan (who had an office in the hotel) was re-elected in a landslide, when America was in the throes of a new era of opulence. In 2000, following a US$43 million renovation and re-branding, the hotel left its '80s chintz and gilding behind and re-emerged as a charming spot for the new millennium — and one with a spa that caters to some of the most influential faces of our times.

LOCATION

The 297-room hotel and spa is a bull's eye for the city centre, located in the heart of Century City on L.A.'s hoity-toity Westside. It's a mile from Beverly Hills and about ten minutes to Santa Monica and downtown. The MGM and Fox studios are right across the street, while Century City Shopping Center, the city's best outdoor mall, is just around the corner. In a town infamous for freeway gridlock, this easy-to-get-to-and-go-from locale makes the St. Regis the hotel of choice for A-list road-ragers, as well as the setting for events like movie press junkets.

DESIGN

The emphasis is on luxury and elegance, minus the frou-frou, which translates into an intimate and welcoming environment. Rooms are done up in rich woods, French toile and sunny balconies with panoramic views of smoggy Los Angeles. The pool area is Hollywood gorgeous, complete with cabanas and secret gardens. The fitness facility has all the best equipment, including a circuit of seven Cybex machines, and a semicircular wall of floor-to-ceiling windows that looks out onto the pool, as well as Santa Monica and beyond it the Pacific Ocean. The spa has eight multipurpose treatment rooms and the famed Yamaguchi Salon (home of the $250 Billy Yamaguchi haircut), as well as eucalyptus steam room and dry sauna. The relaxation room incorporates the traditional California style of cotton couches and ottomans, local art and cool colours of opally greens and sand. It's what you would imagine Jennifer Aniston's den looking like. The treatment rooms are lovelier than most — the white marble and spaciousness of the hotel's bathrooms carries through.

CLIENTELE

The St. Regis has hosted all U.S. presidents since its first guest, Ronald Reagan, as well as many dignitaries and starlets. Ricky Martin was at the table beside us at breakfast one morning, while Charlize Theron, whose skin was luminous at the Golden Globe Awards the night before, is a regular at the spa. Aesthetician Mia says she routinely gives facials to a plethora of pampered kings, presidents and sports heroes.

TREATMENTS

The high-end Själ skin care line (used by celebs like Sarah Jessica Parker and P. Diddy) have scents like orange flower water and chocolate, contain about fifty active ingredients, minerals and crushed pearls, and are very expensive (US$150–$210 for tiny jars, but just a little dab'll do ya). The Cold Fusion Energy Facial involves about a million enjoyable steps (and a couple that are none-too-enjoyable) designed to exfoliate, oxygenate, hydrate and firm the skin through the use of one's own energy. It begins with a hydrating treatment using magnetized copper and geranium water, followed by a honey-based deep-cleaning mask, then seaweed and algae oil and French clay, an oxygenating citric peel to remove errant cells, and an illuminating serum mist and moisturizer. Also incorporated are a couple more masks, two more peels, a galvanic machine, the dreaded extractions, a face vacuum (a first for me), hot stone foot massage, foot moisturizing and massage, a shoulder and spine massage, and a crystallized spritz and fizz at the end. "You won't have to moisturize for two days," says Mia as I stagger to the door.

FOOD & DRINK

Because of its proximity to Fox and MGM, the St. Regis's signature restaurant, Encore, is one of the city's top spots for the famed L.A. "power breakfast." Looking around the room, you'll never see so many expensive suits tucking into chicken sausage and scrambled eggs. She's a beauty, though: high ceilings and garden views, all done up in a colonial/modern California look of olives, yellows, hardwood and mini palm trees. Named one of *Esquire's* best new restaurants in 2001, signature dishes include Pacific Ono with minted saffron couscous and foamed mango sauce, and lemon pistachio-crusted rack of lamb.

SERVICE

Mia, a long-standing pro in the aesthetics biz, is well known throughout California. She has given her perfect facials to a Rolodex of famous faces (no names, please) and her personality, along with her knowledge and skill, are what set her apart: "Many of my clients call me Mama Mia." She even had a hand in developing the spa's brand new line of exclusive Själ skin care treatments, an alliance that makes the St. Regis a Själ destination spa.

BOTTOM LINE

If you're in L.A, you might as well do it up and do it up right. Stay in swank surroundings, shop at Fred Segal and Barney's, eat at the "it" spots and definitely partake of the best facial that money can buy. With those Själ-minimized pores and glowing skin, you'll be ready for your close-up.

INFORMATION

The St. Regis Spa. 2055 Avenue of the Stars, Los Angeles, CA.. Phone: (310) 277-6111. Web: http://www.stregis.com.
 The Cold Fusion Energy Facial lasts around 50 minutes and costs US$160.

SPATOPIA

THE RITZ-CARLTON HUNTINGTON HOTEL AND SPA, PASADENA

At first glance, Pasadena suggests a city centred around conferences, conventions and Rose Bowl parades. But it's about so much more. Think of exclusive neighbourhoods and charming Old Pasadena. There are museums and playhouses, excellent restaurants and shopping. Plus, spa culture is booming here, especially at the Ritz-Carlton Huntington Hotel and Spa, where you can experience everything from a massage under a willow tree to a tai chi class in the breezy Japanese garden. Even so, I defy you to find someone who hasn't been on convention in Pasadena.

LOCATION

The massive hotel complex is nestled amongst twenty-three acres of gardens and grounds at the foothills of the San Gabriel Mountains, just twenty minutes from downtown Los Angeles. It's about forty-five minutes from Beverly Hills, ten from the Rose Bowl (home to the UCLA Bruins and the annual Rose Bowl game) and under an hour from such Southern Californian favourites as Universal Studios, Disneyland, Hollywood and the beach.

DESIGN

The tree-lined entranceway with its twinkling lights says, "Hello, *dah*-ling," and once inside, the famous Ritz elegance permeates the décor: dark woods and marble, smoky taupe and chandeliers, turn-of-the-century splendour replete with magical gardens and bridges, elegant ballrooms, swimming pool and restaurants. The Ritz-Carlton Huntington Hotel & Spa has almost 400 guest rooms and suites; in addition, separate from the main building are seven bungalows, the Lanai Building, Royce Manor and Clara Vista, which offer a more residential feel. Set amidst it all is more than 2,780 square metres of function space.

The spa is separate from the main property, housed in a former carriage house, so there's a bit of a horsy theme. But it's a 115-square-metre offering of seventeen treatment rooms, the holy trinity of eucalyptus steam room, sauna and whirlpool, plus a state-of-the-art fitness centre and a daily program of exercise classes. In the relaxation room there's dim lighting; candles flickering here and there combine with the dark wood to evoke an old-world feel. Treatment rooms are also quite pretty, tweaked by Californian yellow-and-white-striped walls.

SPAtopia

CLIENTELE

A big spot for weddings and other big gatherings (there was a Water Contamination Conference in house on this day). Many attendees frequent the spa, fitness room and classes during their downtime. Vacations see golf widows and widowers enjoying all-day spa affairs (there are five championship golf courses within twenty minutes of the hotel), but the core clientele are the local spa-sters — fancy ladies here for massages and colour rinses in the salon.

TREATMENTS

When a spa is this big and your regulars this knowledgeable, you've got to be up on the latest thing and serve it up. So, you've got your Ayurvedic treatments, Chinese five-element treatments, violet clay envelopment and the whole gamut of massages. Posh services like the Champagne Facial utilize Champagne yeast extracts from the Champagne region of France (read: none of that mediocre sparkling wine nonsense), combined with exotic Chinese herbs. It's all meant to stimulate and nourish the skin while waging war against free radicals.

The Aromatherapy Hair and Scalp Treatment takes place in a salon chair. Using Aveda oils, Jerrod massages a custom blend of pure flower and plant essence over the neck and into the scalp through a deep massage. You'll start out amicably chatting, but find yourself quickly devolving to incoherent mumbling and, finally, open-mouthed drooling. The oils deliver calming and balancing benefits to all hair types while the aromatherapy component helps relieve stress while invigorating and restoring balance to mind and body. And there is nothing more relaxing than a deep scalp massage. A final lashing of warm oil saturates the hair, then it's under the dryer for ten minutes to let it sink in. A big rinse, shampoo and leave-in conditioner complete the deal. Alberto VO5, eat your heart out.

SERVICE

"First we make the world revolve around you. Then we gently slow it down," says the Ritz's spa brochure in fancy script. Such power! In the salon, Jerrod had strong massage hands and a gentle demeanour.

BOTTOM LINE

If you've got to go to Pasadena for a convention anyway, you might as well take in an aerobics class or have a massage at the spa and make it more of a true vacation. After all, all work and no play makes Jim a dull boy.

INFORMATION

The Ritz-Carlton Huntington Hotel & Spa. 1401 South Oak Knoll Avenue, Pasadena, CA. Phone: (626) 585-6414. Web: http://www.ritzcarlton.com/hotels/huntington/.
The Aromatherapy Hair & Scalp treatment lasts around 55 minutes and costs US$70, including 18 percent gratuity.

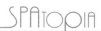

LAS VEGAS SPAS

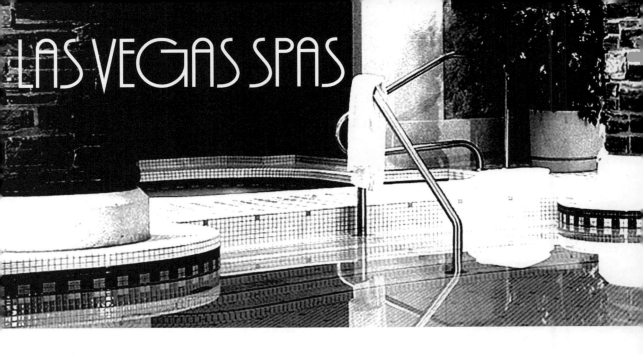

as Vegas is the kind of place you have to see to believe, and even then you don't quite believe it. For half a century up until the early 1990s, the city was widely acknowledged as a Disneyland for adults, a place for hosting raunchy stags, gambling weekends and quickie marriages.

But then Vegas went through an extensive and expensive metamorphosis, whereupon this once X-rated town gained a respectable G rating. Suddenly, Vegas wasn't just for crapshooters and crap-talkers anymore. Everyone was invited.

From Grandpa staked out at the one-armed bandits to a bevy of bridesmaids having group paraffin manicures at a day spa, the new-and-improved Vegas is a place where blackjack takes a back seat, but hedonism still reigns supreme — especially in its many luxurious spas.

LOCATION

A kaleidoscopic oasis carved out of the Nevada desert, the infamous Strip is the six-kilometre stretch of Las Vegas Boulevard between Russell Road and Sahara Avenue. The majority of the city's most opulent spas are located here.

The southern end of the Strip has benefited most from the recent billion-dollar boom, with the opening of hotels such as the kid-friendly New York-New York, the couples-friendly Mandalay Bay and the wealth-friendly Venetian and Bellagio. At the core of the Strip are two classic holdouts: the Flamingo Las Vegas (a mainstay since 1946) and Caesars Palace, which for twenty-five years was the ritziest game in town.

TREATMENTS

Instead of throwing your money away at the blackjack tables, put those greenbacks to good use with a decadent spa treatment at one of Vegas's new high-end spas.

The Passage to India treatment at the **Spa at Caesars Palace** (home to twenty-eight treatment rooms) is based on Ayurvedic rituals from India that combine herb-infused oils and massage to rejuvenate the body and mind. You begin by filling out a Tara Ayurveda Constitutional Analysis so the staff can deduce whether your Tara sign is *vata* (ether and air), *pitta* (fire and water) or *kapha* (water and earth). Your aesthetician (ask for Nanette) then mixes together a personal herb combo based on your sign. The 120 minutes of various body masks and deep-tissue massage (among other things) ends with a thick application of infused oil and a drink of herb-infused tea. You leave looking and feeling like a more peaceful you.

The **Canyon Ranch SpaClub**, housed in the romantic Venetian hotel (with its whitewashed walls and network of canals and gondoliers) is a gorgeous nugget that has been frequented by such luminaries as Kirsten Dunst and Cindy Crawford. Treatments range from massage therapies and fitness training to signature services such as Canyon Stone Massage and Body Cocoons. Private rooms can be had for a group stagette manicure session topped off by warm paraffin wax. Very *Sex and the City*.

To truly get away from it all, hit the **Four Seasons**, the only hotel on the strip without a casino. Its ethereal sixteen-treatment-room spa is equally unique, featuring Asian rituals and Balinese treatments such as the Balinese foot wash, which kicks off with a warm, flower-scented foot bath followed by exfoliation using volcanic clay, then a revitalizing foot massage.

FOOD & DRINK

Vegas has evolved from being dominated by rib-roast and all-you-can-eat shrimp buffets to a gourmand's dream. Many U.S. celebrity chefs, such as Emeril, Wolfgang Puck and Todd English, have opened at least one satellite restaurant here.

Mr. Puck's Spago, located in the Forum Shops of Caesars Palace, is just a few escalator rides from the Caesars spa and serves crisp calamari with orange basil aioli, famous wood-fired salmon pizza and desserts so decadent they could only be served in Sin City.

Better still, plan your spa treatments to coincide with tea time. High tea at the Four Seasons sees a pianist tickling the ivories as the open French doors of the Verandah Lounge usher in warm desert breezes. Then comes fine bone china filled with custom-blended loose teas, dainty sandwiches — such as prosciutto with fig and port cream cheese — and assorted tarts, scones and chocolates.

BOTTOM LINE

You need only go once, but do go to Vegas before you die — if only to experience the Passage to India treatment.

INFORMATION

Caesars Palace. 3570 Las Vegas Boulevard South, Las Vegas, NV. Phone: 1-877-427-7243. Web: http://www.caesars.com/caesars/lasvegas. For bookings at the spa and salon call (702) 731-7776. The Passage to India treatment costs US$250.

Canyon Ranch SpaClub. 3355 Las Vegas Boulevard South, Las Vegas, NV.
Phone: (702) 414-3600 or 1-877-220-2688.
Web: http://www.canyonranch.com/spaclubs/venetian.
The Spa Manicure costs US$45, plus $20 for paraffin treatment.

Spago (located in the Forum Shops at Caesars Palace). 3500 Las Vegas Boulevard South, Las Vegas, NV.
Phone: (702) 369-6300. Web: http://www.wolfgangpuck.com.

Spa at the Four Seasons Hotel Las Vegas. 3960 Las Vegas Boulevard South, Las Vegas. NV. Phone: (702) 632-5302. Web: http://www.fourseasons.com/lasvegas. The Balinese Foot Wash is US$75. Afternoon tea is served from 2 p.m. to 5 p.m. for $21 a person.

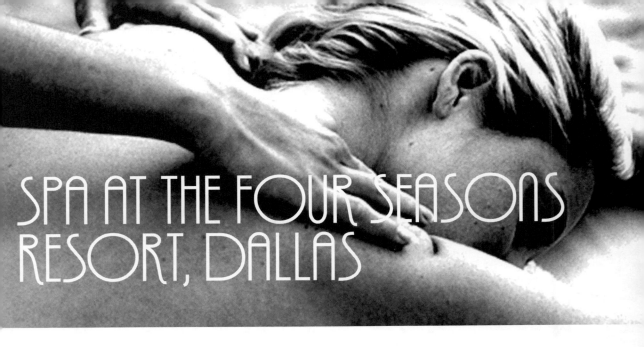

SPA AT THE FOUR SEASONS RESORT, DALLAS

Texas is all about membership. You wear your university colours with pride, then buy your monster home in the right part of town. You belong to a golf club and private cigar bar, sit on several boards and committees and frequent the same steak house, which houses your own private wine locker. It's all about going big or going home, which is why the salon and spa at the Four Seasons Resort and Club in Dallas is such a welcome respite for harried social climbers. This is where business comes to work out — and then settle down.

LOCATION

A perfectly manicured North Texas landscape of mesquite trees, gentle knolls and sand dunes, set amidst 160 hectares of the Tournament Players Club golf course. The wealthiest of the wealthy (oilmen, former high-tech whiz kids and professional athletes) have built their enormous homes overlooking these emerald greens. The resort is a fifteen-minute drive from the Dallas/Fort Worth International Airport, half an hour from downtown Dallas, and smack-dab in the middle of the upscale community of Las Colinas. Texas Stadium (home to the Dallas Cowboys since 1971) is a five-minute drive away, and the flagship Neiman Marcus department store is twenty minutes distant, as is the American Airlines Center, home to the NBA's Dallas Mavericks — more than a few of whom frequent the Four Seasons spa.

DESIGN

The resort's 357 rooms, suites and villas are a study in understated elegance, all with balconies, views, marble bathrooms and guaranteed good sleeps in those trademark beds with oversized feather pillows.

The spa, on the other hand, is looking a little long in the tooth. It's large and open, clean and well kept. But this place was designed when Pat Benatar and Spandau Ballet were atop the charts; the outdated peaches-and-greens colour scheme and faux weathered wrought-iron accents look more like a Florida sunroom than Four Seasons chic. Happily, the spa was recently slated for a major renovation and will no doubt emerge as a fashionable phoenix.

CLIENTELE

This is no typical Four Seasons resort, in that many of the guests walking about are Sports Club members, meaning they come almost daily to play tennis and tee off, enroll the kids in swimming lessons, and take yoga and spinning classes. And you can bet that more than a few deals have been hatched over drinks at the pool cabana. There are two championship eighteen-hole golf courses (one being the home of the annual PGA Tour's Byron Nelson Championship), a 3,000-square-metre conference centre, a 750-square-metre ballroom and a 550-square-metre fitness centre.

One can only imagine the numbers of wedding guests and meeting-goers vying for an appointment at the salon or sports massage at the spa. But in fact, area residents who aren't club members make up the main portion of spa habitués (about 40 percent), with resort guests a close second, followed by club members getting in on that cactus contouring body-glaze action.

TREATMENTS

The Texan Two-Step treatment is so branded for two reasons: it's divided into two distinct steps, obviously, but also because the idea is that you'll be so sprightly and loose afterwards that you'll be raring to dance. The treatment starts off in the usual way: naked under a towel in a white-tiled room. The body is rubbed with oil, and then a blue-corn body polish (corn meal ground to a semi-fine dust) is applied with friction, front and back, to nourish the skin with oil while sloughing away dead cells. Shower off, change rooms, and it's time for an hour-long Swedish massage, which uses an oil based on indigenous sagebrush (akin to eucalyptus), a traditional herbal medicine that's meant to relieve muscle soreness and aid circulation. "Growing up, I remember my mother would grind it with alcohol and soak her feet in it to soothe them after work," says my Mexican massage therapist, Mary.

The spa has an extensive roster of treatments, ranging from hot-stone massages and paraffin body wraps to travellers' relief baths and detoxifying pumpkin-enzyme facials. Heading from the West to the Pacific, the Fiji pedicure, with therapist Dee Dee, involves an hour of delicious foot fetishism. Feet are bathed in a coconut milk bath, exfoliated with a sugar scrub, massaged with nut oil, rubbed with thick coconut butter and wrapped in steamed towels, then the nails are painted. With your feet smelling good enough to eat, the spa has wisely included a coconut fruit smoothie to go with the treatment.

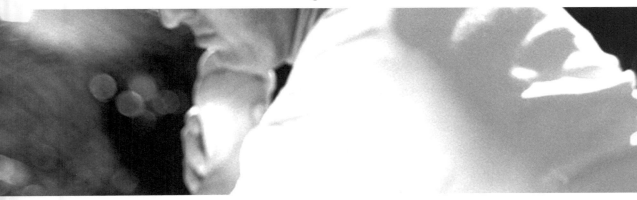

FOOD & DRINK

The resort has several good restaurants. An après-golf lunch can be had at Byron's by the first fairway, or have a snack at Racquets after creaming your tennis partner. Classy cocktails can be consumed at the Terrace Lounge, and formal room service is always an option. But best is Café on the Green, which dishes up new American vittles tweaked by Asian influences. The room itself is gorgeous, the décor reminiscent of a colonial Japanese bistro (if that's possible). Smoked ancho chili-and-red-pepper amuse-bouche sips set the tone, curried mango-and-orange soup with lump crabmeat is refreshingly light, and braised barbecue beef ribs with garlic mash and Asian slaw remind you that you're in cowboy country.

Nutritionally balanced selections of healthier gourmet fare, such as soy-marinated salmon sashimi, crispy tofu with vegetables and shiitake–star anise glaze — is also deliciously (and non-sinfully) on offer at all resort dining venues.

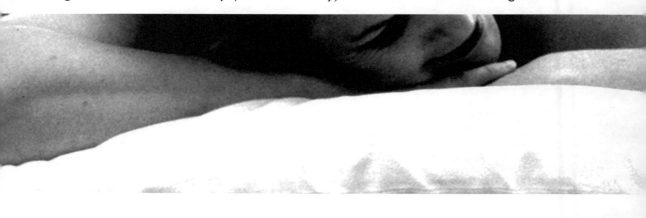

SERVICE

Staff members call you "Ms.," and most have Southern accents, which is fun. And that Mary sure knows her way around a Texan two-step.

BOTTOM LINE

From car dealers attending a conference to tourists reclining by the pool, this may not be a members-only resort, but they sure make you feel like you belong. After a few hours at the Four Seasons spa you'll be raring to take on a bull market — or a mechanical bull. Take your pick.

INFORMATION

Four Seasons Resort and Club at Las Colinas. 4150 North MacArthur Boulevard, Irving, TX. Phone: 1-800-332-3442 or (972) 717-0700.
Web: http://www.fourseasons.com/dallas.
The Texas Two-Step lasts 90 minutes and costs US$195. The Fiji pedicure is an hour long, costs $70, and includes a yummy smoothie.

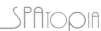

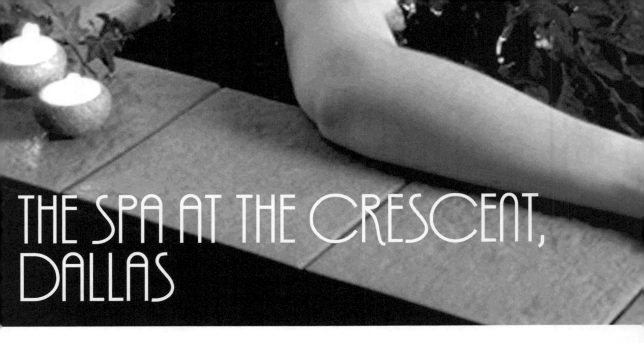

THE SPA AT THE CRESCENT, DALLAS

There's no denying that spa treatments with kitschy names are guaranteed to win over the spa habitué — and punster, for that matter — every time. After all, why have a plain old stone massage when you can experience a Hotter 'n' Texas Summer Rock Massage?

With close to eighty original treatments, the Spa at the Crescent has amassed a roster of real knee-slappers that will pique the interest, mollify the body — and maybe even tantalize the taste buds. Texas-Style Barbecue Body Experience, anyone?

LOCATION

This curvaceous jumble of modern, château-style buildings is anchored by a mixed-use development that includes three eighteen-storey office towers, restaurants and shops, the Crescent Hotel, and its spa. Situated in Dallas's wonderful downtown Arts District, it's just a five-minute drive to the central business district (you could walk it in fifteen, but nobody walks in Dallas), the Dallas Market Center and one of the most affluent residential areas in the state.

DESIGN

The spa and fitness centre recently underwent a US$4 million renovation, but even so, the décor is a touch passé, with its colour palate of creams and sage, live ferns, and tilework with old-school Southwestern flair. The upper-level workout area is Texas-sized, while the comfy lounge area has the casual feel of someone's home. The TV even shows the afternoon soaps. There's also a separate men's area, sixteen treatment rooms, the water works — steam room, sauna, whirlpool and pool — and salon and pedicure stations.

The Juice Bar is light and airy, with marble bistro tables and bevelled mirrors. Fortified smoothies, such as the Tower of Power, are served alongside delicious low-fat spa cuisine with Tex-Mex flair — spinach and mushroom enchiladas with roasted tomatillo sauce and black bean succotash, for example.

In the large locker room, the post-treatment staging area — where one spruces up before heading back into the world — is a little larger and more gilded than most, and comes stocked with lotions, hairspray, hot rollers and curling irons. Lest we forget, this is Big Hair Country.

CLIENTELE

Everyone from friends with Louis Vuitton totes just here for the day, to metro-sexuals working out in the gym before getting a specialty Kur treatment in the spa.

In the Juice Bar, a distinguished man in a terry-cloth robe — who looks vaguely familiar — is obviously a regular but today is being greeted with "Congratulations!" and "That's absolutely incredible!" A look at the front page of the *Dallas Morning News* makes it apparent who he is: the day before, this surgeon spent thirty-three hours successfully separating two Egyptian boys joined at the head. If this guy doesn't deserve a day at the spa, nobody does.

TREATMENTS

After hoofing around in pointy-toed boots all day, the Cowboy Boogie might be just the ticket for those aching dogs. Perched atop a massaging pedicure throne, you soak in the whirlpool foot bath to loosen cuticles while a heated sack soothes the neck. Steve sands down the heels, dries off the feet, then slops on mineral-rich moor mud, after which the feet are wrapped in plastic and placed in heated booties. (Sometimes things have to get ugly before they can get pretty.)

After ten minutes the mud is removed and the old nail polish comes off. Cuticles and nails get snipped and shaped, then comes a sugar scrub and a pumice-stone treatment (for those stubborn spots). Oil is mixed with lavender cream, and legs and feet get a deep massage. Nails get a base coat, a couple of coats of polish and a top coat — and you're ready to dance the two-step.

The Texas Crushed Cabernet Body Scrub takes its cues from newly popular vinotherapy treatments which use grape byproducts (in this case, seeds and peels from Napa cabernet grapes) to scrub and strengthen skin by protecting it from free radicals. Grape byproducts are high in OPCs (oligomeric proantho-cyanidins), antioxidants said to be more potent than vitamins C and E.

In a wet room, Rick douses the body with a Scotch hose, then works in the exfoliating mixture limb by limb before rinsing it off with a loofah sponge and the hose. Dry off, change rooms, and then it's a candlelit massage using soothing lavender cream.

SERVICE

Joyce works the crowds in the locker room, showing everyone what's what and where's where; doling out loaned gym outfits, ice-cold eucalyptus face towels, ginger-peach herbal tea, fresh fruit cups and good cheer. Rick is all business as he scrubs and massages, while Steve's pedicure shows master craftsmanship.

BOTTOM LINE

The treatments are so relaxing you might acquire a drawl — and that's not just whistling Dixie. The Spa at the Crescent earned the distinction of Top Urban Spa in North America from *Condé Nast Traveler* in 2002, as well as a mention in its list of Top Five Spas for Treatments.

INFORMATION

The Spa at the Crescent. 400 Crescent Court, Dallas, TX. Phone: (214) 871-3232. Web: http://www.crescentcourt.com/spa.cfm. The Texas Crushed Cabernet Body Scrub lasts 50 minutes and costs US$95; the Cowboy Boogie also lasts 50 minutes and costs $75.

SPATOPIA

THE SPA AT THE FOUR SEASONS HOTEL, CHICAGO

If you were to scout locations for the "fancy lobby scene" of a big-budget film, the sizable marble fountain, brocade armchairs and flower-filled entrance of the sixty-six-storey Four Seasons Hotel Chicago would fit the bill. It's all about big welcomes and in-your-face opulence.

But you've got to do more than just smile and look pretty to earn both the 2002 Mobil Five-Star and the 2002 AAA Five Diamond awards, the hotel industry's highest honours. Could it be their famously comfy beds? The fabulous shopping on Chicago's adjacent Magnificent Mile? The concierge-arranged *Oprah* tickets?

Suave service, great location and luxe surroundings are what set a premier hotel apart from a merely great hotel. Did we mention the multimillion-dollar spa and fitness centre, which just won the *Condé Nast Traveler* award for top hotel spa in North America?

LOCATION

From the ashes of the Great Chicago Fire of 1871 emerged an architecturally gifted city (this is the birthplace of the modern skyscraper) that showcases the works of such masters as Frank Lloyd Wright and Ludwig Mies van der Rohe, as well as many thoughtful promenades and downtown plazas.

Right outside the hotel is Michigan Avenue, also known as the Magnificent Mile, the jumping-off point for any legitimate shopping spree. It's where you'll find Burberry, Chanel, Gucci and Saks Fifth Avenue. Veering off North Michigan Avenue, you'll find an exquisite oasis of calm in the tree-lined area known as the Gold Coast. On Oak Street, which is akin to Toronto's Yorkville, there is a mix of upscale designers (Prada, Sonia Rykiel), specialty stores and fine dining. Within ten minutes of the hotel is the Lincoln Park Zoo, with fourteen child-friendly hectares of animals, birds and reptiles. Also within striking distance are the must-see Museum of Contemporary Art and the John Hancock Center, with its ninety-fourth-floor observatory offering a bird's-eye view of Lake Michigan, the city skyline and, when skies are clear, four different states.

DESIGN

A sumptuous explosion of chandeliers, loomed textiles and carpeting, marble, brass, burnished leather and rich wood panelling and chinoiserie. In the spa lounge, daybeds fill niches with overstuffed silk pillows.

CLIENTELE

When you're paying US$400 a night on average for a room, you can expect to see plenty of lap dogs.

SPATOPIA

TREATMENTS

In August 2001, the hotel unveiled its fitness centre with a new spa, featuring five soundproof treatment rooms outfitted in Frette linen, an aesthetics room for nail treatments and a spa lounge laden with refreshing elixirs, daybeds and patrons so relaxed you'd think they were in comas. The expanded fitness centre has the full range of cardiovascular machines, weight-training equipment, Roman column–flanked swimming pool, whirlpool and steam rooms.

But it's the spa that has attracted some of the best aestheticians in the biz. The signature service is an odourless Perle de Caviar Facial — rich in omega-3 fatty acids, iron and vitamins A, E and K. Pearl proteins and moisturizing marine agents take action in the form of creams, scrubs, massages and masks to firm and revitalize a particularly parched visage. After the fifty-minute treatment, shuffle over to the relaxation room for more caviar; this time, beluga eggs on toast points with a split of Chandon champagne. The spa offers a full range of popular and unique treatments, including a Gentlemen's Urban Defense Facial, enzyme peels, crushed pearl and lavender body polish and green tea and ginger mud mask.

FOOD & DRINK

The spa cuisine has been designed by executive chef Mark Baker, and entrees (all $18) are available before or after treatments in the spa lounge. Choose from the likes of organic farmhouse greens with rosemary-grilled chicken breast, or sesame-seared ahi tuna with pea greens and bean-sprout salad. Food snobbery hits a new high with their "carpaccio of seasonal fruits," more commonly known as fruit salad.

If spa food isn't your thing, Chicago is a great restaurant town, and an even better snack city. Dive into the deep-dish pies at Gino's Pizza (on Rush Street) or the freshly made kettle-cooked chips at Corner Bakery (found at several locations throughout the city). The lineup for homemade caramel corn at Garrett's on Michigan Avenue often snakes around the corner.

The Four Seasons' Sunday brunch is an annual winner of the Zagat Chicago Survey's "top brunch spot." Six international food stations offer Peking duck, rack of lamb, seared tuna, shrimp cocktail, homemade granola, crème brûlé, fresh omelettes and crepes. With more choices than you can shake a fork at, the superb service and courtly décor simply become excellent extras.

SERVICE

Professional and accommodating. Some lack a sense of humour, while others happily thumb their noses at the whole snobbery trip. If you can, book spa treatments with head aesthetician Florica. She's informative and funny and has magic hands.

BOTTOM LINE

This is the Four Seasons, after all. Expect the best, then be pleasantly surprised.

INFORMATION

Four Seasons Hotel Chicago. 120 East Delaware Place, Chicago, Il. Phone: 1-800-268-6282. Web: www.fourseasons.com/chicagofs. Spa reservations: (312) 280-8800 ext. 2174. Book treatments well ahead of your visit as they often sell out, especially on weekends. Spa appointments from 8 a.m.–8 p.m. In-room spa services available for an additional surcharge of 25 percent. Four Seasons Perle de Caviar facial costs US$65 for 30 minutes, $110 for 50 minutes, $155 for 80 minutes. Fitness Centre open 6 a.m.–11 p.m. daily. Brunch is served Sundays 10:30 a.m.–1:30p.m. Reserve at (312) 649-2349.

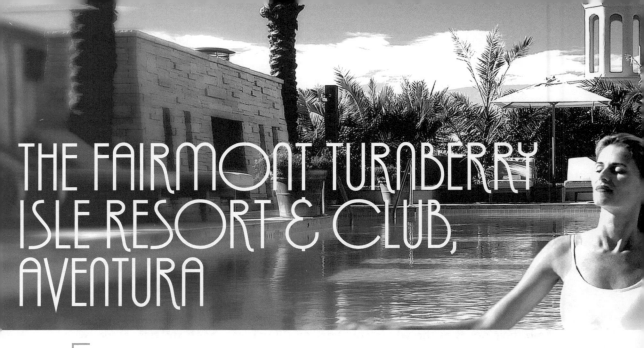

THE FAIRMONT TURNBERRY ISLE RESORT & CLUB, AVENTURA

Even though the heyday of the aged industrialist and his trophy wife has long since passed, there's a back-to-the-future trend afoot as exclusive golf and country clubs across North America are on the upswing. It all goes along with the new bourbon, beef and Boxster lifestyle, a luxurious echo of simpler times.

And although it is members-only, the spa at the Turnberry Isle Resort & Club isn't as elitist as it might seem. Instead of marrying up and paying thousands in initiation fees, all you really need to gain entry into this inner sanctum is a registered room key. The newly rebranded (as of January 30, 2004) Fairmont property is a Mediterranean-style resort with championship golf courses, two tennis clubs, multiple restaurants, the 2,300-square-metre spa and fitness centre, a marina and the private Ocean Club.

LOCATION

Aventura is a wealthy enclave in North Miami (a midway point between Fort Lauderdale and South Beach), and the Turnberry has been a fixture in these exclusive parts since the 1970s. The resort is within walking distance of the massive Aventura Mall (Bloomingdale's, Macy's and 248 other stores) and a short drive to the Bal Harbour Shops (a ritzy step up with Neiman Marcus and Saks Fifth Avenue). Pro Player Stadium (home turf for the Miami Dolphins and Florida Marlins) and American Airlines Arena (which houses the NBA's Miami Heat) are also nearby, as are the Office Depot Center (the NHL's Florida Panthers), Hialeah and Calder Race Courses, Hollywood and Biscayne Dog Tracks, and the Tennis Center at Key Biscayne.

DESIGN

The great hotels of Europe inspired the overall look of the resort, and that translates into a classical architectural style of pillars, promenades and terra cotta roofs. The spa, which was christened a Willow Stream Spa in April 2004 (a change that was to entail some menu and cosmetic changes), is three-tiered and anchored by a lovely spiral staircase that winds around a waterfall and fountain. The spacious relaxation area is gender neutral and comes fortified with a row of the most powerful massage loungers known to man. The twenty-six treatment rooms are painted in watery greens and blues with light hardwood floors, while the mango-scented steam room, shower and makeup areas are tarted up with bright turquoise tile work.

SERVICE

Everyone seems to have been trained in that warm, "How can we help you" Fairmont style. Massage therapist Vonnie was the perfect mix of spiritual guide ("This is your special time"), fun pal ("Wow, doesn't it smell great in here?") and hands-on healer.

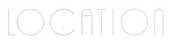

SPATOPIA

120

AMY ROSEN

CLIENTELE

You must be a guest of the resort or a member of the club to gain entrance to the spa and health club, but that can include everyone from incentive groups, which sometimes take over the entire spa, to golf pros, tons of retired locals, and vacationing sun worshippers and spa habitués.

TREATMENTS

The spa at the Turnberry has a superb roster of treatments, both high tech and down home, on offer. For example, Sound Therapy, which uses Crystal Singing Bowls. In theory, the sounds emanating from the bowls can release blockages, allowing energy to flow through the body. There's also the Samadhi Mud Ceremony, an ancient Middle Eastern journey that can be shared with friends in the spa's own Samadhi Room. Or how about the Glycolic Acid Treatment — organic alpha hydroxyl acids designed to even skin pigmentation damage as well as soften fine lines. But best are the rituals, which incorporate the techniques, products and spirit of their namesake geographical regions, be they Ayurvedic, Balinese, Thai, or the new Aboriginal rituals.

This spa was the first to bring the Aboriginal rituals and products to the United States. The Dreaming Body Ritual involves indigenous products harvested by Australian Aboriginal tribes who believe that certain fruits and herbs restore and heal the body, and that traditions like smudging (whereby incense is burned in a pretty little bowl and floated around the body to open you up to what you're about to receive) are just as important as a deep-tissue massage.

You lose yourself in about 1,001 steps that fuse the indigenous medicines and massage techniques with aromatherapy, colour therapy and herbalist principles. Various types of body massage, mini-facial, hair masque, hand and foot treatments, mud wrap and steam, all using techniques from the Australian Aboriginal tribes. The products are especially interesting, like macadamia facial cream (macadamias contain mainly monounsaturated fat, which is the closest to the skin's natural sebum); purifying kelp and clay masque (the high iodine content stimulates circulation, aiding in the cleansing and revitalizing process); wattleseed protein polish (has a high protein and carbohydrate content and acts as a physical and enzyme-action exfoliant); quandong hair masque (the quandong has long been used by Aboriginal peoples to enrich the lustre of their hair); and chokerre mapi (active Australian clay rich in minerals like silica, magnesium, potassium, calcium, iron and zinc). It's like going to the Outback, minus the twenty-four-hour flight.

BOTTOM LINE

In these fast-paced times the ritual — be it historical, philosophical, spiritual, or all of the above — is a dying art. Leave it to a spa to reconnect you with the time-honoured traditions of Australia's Aboriginal tribes. Go in for a Dreaming Body Ritual and come though the other side an expert on *Li'Tya* ("of the earth"). Or, at the very least, leave with some inside knowledge of the secret ingredients that keep those tribe elders' skin so silky soft.

INFORMATION

Fairmont Turnberry Isle Resort & Club. 19999 West Country Club Drive, Aventura, FL.
Phone: (305) 932-6200 or 1-800-327-7028.
Web: http://www.fairmont.com/turnberryisle.
The Dreaming Body Ritual lasts 110 minutes and costs US$279.

SPATOPIA

DORAL GOLF RESORT & SPA, MIAMI

The sunny climes of Miami have long been a favourite destination for silver-haired snowbirds seeking to escape the harsh realities of our Canadian winters. And until recently that has meant golf, discount shopping, early-bird specials and more golf. But times have changed and Florida has changed right along with them. From a rejuvenated Art Deco district to high-end malls, cutting-edge cuisine and now some of the best spas in the world — this isn't your grandfather's Miami. Which isn't to say that Gramps wouldn't enjoy a nice sports hydro-aromatherapy treatment now and again.

LOCATION

Surrounded by 650 acres of luscious tropics, the Doral is just ten minutes from Miami International Airport, and less than half an hour from the glitz and glam of Coconut Grove, Coral Gables, South Beach, and Bal Harbour Village — home to the legendary Bal Harbour Shops, where the people-watching prospects are on a par with Beverly Hills and St-Tropez.

DESIGN

The Doral is a huge property, featuring five championship golf courses (the site has hosted the PGA Tour since 1962), five restaurants, the Arthur Ashe Tennis Center and the Jim McLean Golf School. The Spa at Doral is on the same grounds, but is serenely separated from the rest of the resort.

"What do you think?" asked the woman next to me in the locker area. She said she had loved her treatments (the spa is routinely ranked one of the best destination spas in the world and was just named one of the top ten spas in America by *Spa Finder Magazine* and the Zagat Survey) but was surprised to find the place looking a bit "weathered." Crooked shower doors, tiles coming off in the spa pool area, ripped robes — the sort of details that are easily avoided, and quite disconcerting when you're paying for the best. That said, much of the spa has been recently renovated, with more fix-ups to come.

The expansive relaxation room is chock full of overstuffed furniture and is as comforting as Granny's condo. The rest of the spa and its lovely grounds are inspired by classic Tuscan villas, with gardens, fountains, pools, balustraded patios and quaint courtyards. The spa has a whopping fifty-two treatment rooms, the Chopra Center (for meditation retreats, yoga and "emotional clearing exercises") and a high-tech exercise centre.

There are forty-eight private spa suites set away from the main golf resort rooms, and they feature big comfy beds, dressing areas, marble bathrooms, Jacuzzis and picture-postcard views of the formal gardens and golf greens.

CLIENTELE

There are "loads of mommies," says aesthetician Barbara. "And younger girls, too. And more and more men are having facials and even body wraps. It's nice to see them finally taking care of themselves." She says elder snowbirds also flock to the spa, some using Doral as a spa destination, others as a golf getaway. Famous folk stop by too, including Cheech Marin (of Cheech and Chong), and Barbara counts the baseball star Roger Clemens and former Vice President Al Gore amongst her private clients. "Gore hasn't been back since he lost the election, though."

TREATMENTS

With more than a hundred treatments to choose from, you can make an hour of it or settle in for a full week of pampering. Selections range from the Blue Monster Massage (a therapeutic salve-based rubdown named after Doral's famed PGA golf course) to teeth whitening and a tarot card reading (of all things!). Best is the spa's new Ayurvedic treatments inspired by the Chopra Center.

Book your Odyssey with Barbara, and you'll come face to face with a 5,000-year-old healing philosophy, specific to your body type (Vita, Pitta or Kapha). You will be massaged, scrubbed, oiled, kneaded, wrapped and rinsed. You will exit the room while Barbara changes the heated massage table, alters the lighting to red and sets up the Shirodhara contraption. Once the bowl of warm oil is strategically placed over your forehead, a gentle but constant stream of sesame oil hits your "third eye" while she rotates it, bringing intuition, relaxation and peace to your being. Sounds like torture, but it's actually a wonderful feeling. "This whole treatment is great for releasing toxins," says Barbara. How so? Through the pores? "Um, not exactly. Some people experience a bit of diarrhea." Oy.

Taking a private class over at the golf school is great for newbies and pros alike; the trained young bucks in fancy pants teach you how to improve your grip, stance and so forth. And zipping around in the golf cart is totally fun.

FOOD & DRINK

There are five on-site restaurants, including the high-end Windows on the Green, which offers such Caribbean-tweaked local specialties as lobster, sautéed shrimp and seasonal stone crab. Terrazza Restaurant and Café has a casual atmosphere and serves up continental fare, a breakfast buffet and Starbucks to go. Champions Sports Bar and Grill offers post-golf grub like club sandwiches, brews and happy hour specials, while the Atrium Restaurant at the Spa goes the opposite route with health-conscious salads and such. Bungalou's Bar & Grill is conveniently located poolside, so you won't have to venture far for those nachos and iced tea.

SERVICE

Barbara calls you "honey" and "sweetie." She's an old-time pro (more than thirty years in the biz), but still takes courses to bone up on the latest trends, like Aboriginal treatments and Shirodhara. Scott at the golf school was an excellent teacher with the patience of a monk.

BOTTOM LINE

Whether you visit the Doral for its world-class spa or for its championship golf courses, it's definitely the best of both worlds. Especially if you book a Shirodhara treatment and get working on that "third eye" business: calming the nervous system, integrating mind and body — and perhaps taking a few strokes off of your golf game as a side benefit.

INFORMATION

Doral Golf Resort and Spa. 4400 NW 87th Avenue, Miami, FL.
Web: http://www.doralresort.com. Phone: (305) 592-2000 or 1-800-71-DORAL.
The Odyssey with Shirodhara treatment lasts 90 minutes and costs US$240. Golf lessons at the Jim McLean Golf School start at $115 per hour. Spa suite rates start at $280.

THE SPA AT THE MANDARIN ORIENTAL, MIAMI

Business travel and luxury accommodations are no longer mutually exclusive now that savvy jet-setters have been turned on to the pleasures of pairing work with play as they ascend the corporate ladder. With its new private beach club and super-luxe spa, the secluded Mandarin Oriental is an elegant antidote to the saucy hot-pants-and-salsa beat of South Beach. Here, guests sip champagne by the infinity pool and pass the time in spa suites — scheduling year-end board meetings in between, of course.

LOCATION

The Mandarin is a quick drive across the causeway from South Beach towards the downtown financial district. The shining hotel is a focal point of the prestigious manmade island of Brickell Key, where you are surrounded by the bluest of waterfront views. Brickell Key (a.k.a. Claughton Island) is a forty-four-acre island in Biscayne Bay, built in 1943 to be one of the city's most prestigious commercial and residential areas. Nearby are all the big bank towers to meet the needs of business travellers, as well as pro sports stadiums and the Bayside Marketplace: 100 shops, thirty restaurants, live music nightly. Also mere moments away are children's favourites, including Parrot Jungle Island, the Miami Seaquarium, Everglades Safari Park and Monkey Jungle.

DESIGN

The 329 guestrooms and suites, pool, beach club, spa and restaurants are all built into the hotel's saucy curved architecture, which, not coincidentally, mimics the Mandarin Hotel Group's fan-shaped logo. From the modern lobby's soaring ceilings and views of Biscayne Bay and the Atlantic Ocean, to the plush rooms with marble bathrooms and top-notch amenities (all of which also afford guests waterfront views), the spa is the elegant knockout. It's a 15,000-square-foot sanctuary of men's and women's relaxation rooms, steams and saunas, yoga studio, and group pedicure area, all of which are done up in blond wood and glass, veined marble floors of light earthen hues, bamboo shutters and cozy cotton chairs with Thai silk pillows and Japanese accents. You'll also find a cutting-edge fitness centre, ten treatment rooms, a hydrotherapy room and six expansive private spa suites. A lovely offshoot of the spa is the hotel's new 20,000-square-foot private, white-sand beach club, with palm trees and beach butlers, stylish oversized snoozing cushions, hammocks and breezy white cabanas for outdoor massages (singles or couples).

CLIENTELE

There are vacationing family groups and amorous couples (mostly European and Asian), but the majority of guests are corporate clients taking advantage of the fifteen meeting/function rooms and the business facilities. One night we witnessed a corporate meet-and-greet where the beach club was decked out in flowers and candles, a private bar, waiter-served noshes and twinkling lights. Little wonder Forbes.com listed it amongst its top eight new business hotels in the world in 2001. At the spa, there was a steady stream of men checking in for massages and facials. Little-known fact: Luciano Pavarotti was the first guest to experience the spa's Oriental Suite.

TREATMENTS

The three-storey spa takes a holistic approach inspired by the ancient traditions of Chinese, Ayurvedic, European, Balinese and Thai cultures; signature treatments include the likes of Thai Massage and Balinese Synchronized Massage. The spa just launched an innovative concept called Time Rituals, in which a grouping of highly personalized treatments are performed in the spa suites and clients are charged by the amount of time they spend in the suite rather than for pre-selected treatments off the à la carte spa menu. My Ayurvedic Holistic Body Treatment took place in a split-level suite on the spa's top floor. All suites feature floor-to-ceiling glass windows and picture-perfect bay views, private shower and deep tub.

The ritual begins with the ringing of Tibetan bells; there are candles and a foot treatment in which the feet are soaked in a petal-scattered basin of warm water doctored with aromatherapy oils. Your feet are massaged while you sip a herbal infusion and, letting your nose be your guide, select the ESPA brand holistic products to be used in your treatment. Next up, a full-body exfoliation scrub, a mini-facial, a clay hair mask, and an intriguing Ayurvedic Marma massage that concentrates on the energy centres of the face and body. This consists of oil-slicked special strokes and some pinpoint accuracy, one side of the body at a time, all meant to release tension and restore vitality. It ends with a chakra head and scalp massage — and a final ringing of the Tibetan bells.

FOOD & DRINK

There are two superb restaurants on site: Café Sambal (named one of America's best by *Gourmet* magazine) and Azul, where the star chef Michelle Bernstein whips up such five-diamond fare as Caribbean Bouillabaisse. Sambal is a modern Asian bistro done up in marble, bamboo and water features, with a wraparound terrace and a stainless-steel sushi bar at the back. Start with iced green tea and complimentary fried wonton chips with a sweet, wasabi-mayo-based dipping sauce, then choose from the delicious selection of "small plates" (for instance, pan-fried chicken dumplings), "large plates" (chilled Florida stone crab claws with miso mustard sauce), salads (Vietnamese shrimp salad) and "bowls and noodles" (pad Thai). There are also spa bento boxes on offer, as well as some of the best sushi in the city (hint: try the Sambal Roll).

SERVICE

Aesthetician Liz was relaxed, informative, smiley and strong. From pre-setting the shower to the perfect temp, to a winning pitch with those Tibetan chimes, you got the feeling that she, too, was getting something spiritual out of the ritual. Throughout the hotel the service was accompanied by a refreshing can-do attitude.

BOTTOM LINE

A good portion of the guests who stay and spa here lodge at a Mandarin hotel wherever business or pleasure takes them around the globe. The place exudes an air of quiet confidence, which is decadently well earned. After all, this is Miami's only hotel to earn the American Automobile Association's top Five Diamond rating, and the spa has garnered awards including best spa in Miami and best spa in America by such magazines as *Self* and *Travel + Leisure*. High praise for a great place.

INFORMATION

Mandarin Oriental Miami. 500 Brickell Key Drive, Miami, FL. Phone: 1-800-526-6566. Web: http://www.mandarinoriental.com. If you're looking for a blowout spa experience, the Ayurvedic Holistic Body Treatment lasts about two hours and costs US$260 plus an 18 percent gratuity that is automatically added to all spa treatments. Time Ritual treatments are $180 per hour, with a two-hour minimum.

NEMACOLIN WOODLANDS RESORT & SPA, FARMINGTON

You first spot the imposing Chateau LaFayette peeking out from green, treed mountains as you take a final turn on Route 40, about ninety minutes southeast of Pittsburgh. Its grandeur is an indication of what you can expect of the rest of Nemacolin Woodlands Resort & Spa. In addition to more than twenty-two treatment rooms at the spa, this self-contained resort, spread over fifty-six hectares, has thirty-six holes of golf on two PGA-rated championship courses, a large equestrian centre, stocked lakes for fly fishing, a ski centre, clay shooting facility, a staffed children's village, excellent shopping and dining and a multimillion-dollar art collection.

In a nutshell, the place is Disneyland for luxury-seeking adults. The resort is the brainchild of Joseph A. Hardy Sr., an American lumber tycoon who bought the dilapidated property in 1987 with hopes of turning it into a deluxe destination for A-list jet-setters. Which might explain the private landing strip out back.

LOCATION

Smack in the midst of the bucolic Laurel Highlands Mountains of western Pennsylvania, the resort is an hour-long flight from Toronto via Air Ontario turbo-prop plane, or a leisurely six-and-a-half-hour drive. Locals in nearby Farmington brag about the "four seasons" in Fayette County, a veritable Shangri-la for nature lovers. There's white-water rafting in the Youghiogheny River Gorge, spelunking in the Laurel Caverns and camping in the Bear Run Nature Reserve. Also in the area are the historic Fort Necessity National Battlefield and the architectural wonders that are Frank Lloyd Wright's Fallingwater and Kentuck Knob.

DESIGN

The resort employs a mishmash of decorating influences that run the gamut from English Tudor and mounted elk heads to the French Renaissance–inspired entrance replete with vaulted ceilings, gilded crystal chandeliers and two-story Palladian windows. Luxurious rooms are large enough to echo, with hoity-toity décor that is all chintz and tassels. Massive marble bathrooms contain deep-dish tubs so large you could drown sitting upright in one.

Outside, a Zen-inspired garden winds along a path, over a footbridge and on toward good health. Inside the spa, it's very feng shui–forward: slate and river rocks, wood and stainless steel, floor-to-ceiling windows — and water, water everywhere. A tinkling stream, a waterfall wall, shimmering lights, a colour scheme born of nature.

CLIENTELE

The majority of the guests look to be wealthy retirees spending a bit of their off-spring's inheritance on the sly, but there's not a man, woman, child or Pfizer convention

SPATOPIA

attendee who could not remain happily entertained here for a few five-star days. Presidents Bill Clinton and George W. Bush apparently enjoyed themselves here, as did Tiger Woods. There are millionaires from Pittsburgh, honeymooners from Washington, best friends from Buffalo, all wrapped in terry-cloth robes, lunching in the Seasons restaurant.

TREATMENTS

The slick gym offers such must-have classes as body sculpting and Pilates. The pool is long and lean, the whirlpool gigantic, the sauna and steam rooms good and steamy. Subterranean treatment rooms are operating at full tilt, so spa services should be reserved when you book your accommodations. Not to be missed are Nemacolin's trademark kurs, a series of 90-minute treatments based on Euro-chic mud, water and massage. The thermal mineral kur starts out friendly enough: introductions, nudity, a cozy cocoon of moor mud and warm towels. Sleep is not out of the question.

Next, a hop into the tub for hydromassage: water fortified with sea salts and essential mineral oils, and workhorse rotating jets akin to the Swiss-flavoured thalassotherapy. The topper comes with a final Swedish massage.

Then there's the hot stone massage, a designer Swedish massage enhanced by smooth basalt stones. The lights are low, a yellow candle flickers in the corner, crystals hang strategically overhead. A vat of stones are heated, then methodically placed on the "third eye" of the forehead, under the toes and everywhere in between. The body is oiled and the kneading of flesh begins. Hot rocks slither along, rotating, warming and massaging in fluid motions.

FOOD & DRINK

There are ten restaurants and eight lounges on the premises, all of which are distinct and well priced. The Chateau's Tea Room may suit the ladies who lunch, while the elegant Lobby Lounge is just the ticket for the ladies who drink. The leathery private cigar bar is the spot for wheeling and dealing, while PJ's is all about ice cream.

The creative cuisine at the ethereal Seasons restaurant uses organic and local ingredients that have been "nutritionally balanced to promote optimum vitality." Lunch typically includes hydrating spor tea, sushi and a Caesar salad draped with seared yellowfin tuna. Dinner might mean a splendid affair at Lautrec, which has the air of a gay Parisian bistro, with dishes that include baked Burgundy snails and lavender-cured rack of lamb. And the wine cellar has 10,000 bottles.

SERVICE

Professional but down home. As the brochure says, "West Coast Attitude, East Coast Latitude."

BOTTOM LINE

Whether it's the peerless spa treatments, a chance meeting with white-tailed deer while horseback riding, or just a night of kicking back with movies and room service, there's a reason for everyone to go.

INFORMATION

Nemacolin Woodlands Resort & Spa. 1001 LaFayette Drive, Farmington, PA. Phone (724) 329-8555 or 1-800-422-2736. Web: http://www.nemacolin.com.
The 275 guestrooms, suites and townhouses all vary in price. Rooms in the Chateau range from US$195–$345 a night; townhouses are $150–$260. The Thermal Mineral Kur is $195; the Hot Stone Massage is $110.

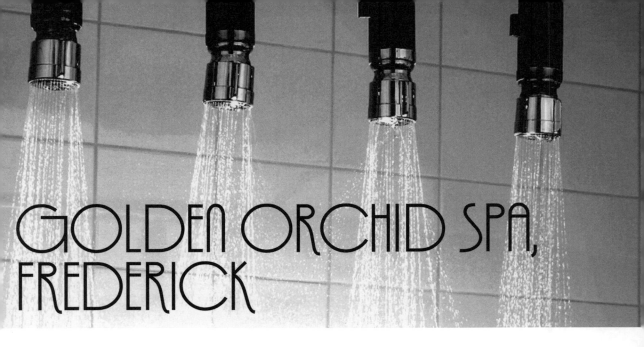

GOLDEN ORCHID SPA, FREDERICK

Just beyond the rolling cornfields, dairy farms and apple orchards of central Maryland is Frederick, a hot spot for Civil War buffs. The city's downtown streets are lined with historic red-brick row houses built in the Federal style, and it is here that Francis Scott Key, author of *The Star-Spangled Banner*, was born and bred.

It is also here that the Golden Orchid Spa set up shop about a year ago in a charming 1800s home. It's an interesting modern-day experience to be surrounded by historical battlefields while taking a soothing afternoon rose-petal soak.

LOCATION

Frederick is located at a crossroads that was witness to modern American history: 72 kilometres northwest of Washington and just 55 kilometres south of Gettysburg. The town's 33-block historic district, with its eighteenth- and nineteenth-century buildings and clustered church spires, is a sweetly inviting cityscape. Walking tours include visits to historic homes, and candlelit ghost tours are also offered.

Market Street, Frederick's main thoroughfare, has dozens of art galleries, bars and restaurants, including Brewer's Alley, which was once the city hall. The Golden Orchid Spa is just off the main strip, behind Shab Row, a newly gentrified antique area that is chock-a-block with cafés and gourmet ice cream shops.

DESIGN

"The house was built in the 1870s," says spa owner Yvette Shirey. "In its first 100 years, ninety-one children were raised here, so it has a lot of life and vitality to it."

And it's got the look and feel of a country inn. "I love to go to B&Bs and inns," she says. "I always want to check out the next one, see what the experience is in a different room. So instead of pigeonholing us into being, say, an Asian spa, I wanted to be able to offer lots of different treatments and emotions that go with the different rooms."

To that end, each room has a different theme, be it celestial, tropical, Asian, Tuscan, or the English garden, where manicures and pedicures are had on the ground floor. The theme here, for example, is reinforced by rose-garden wallpaper, a fireplace, soft greens, hardwood floors and a floral garland around the window, making it feel like a tiny teahouse. It's almost like stopping by the set of *Newhart.*

CLIENTELE

Spa day-trippers plus some spa virgins. Because it has a traditional environment, the Golden Orchid encourages people to take the plunge. Discounts for rebooking mean there are loads of returning locals, plus visitors and groups such as bridal manicure parties who take over the place for an evening.

TREATMENTS

For a small-town spa, it's got some decidedly New Age therapies, including meditation coaching and infant massage groups. Customized facials and other body treatments use the celebrity-approved Bioelements line, which can be custom blended. The product allows aestheticians to add active ingredients to combat issues such as acne or fine lines.

The Golden Orchid's signature spa hand treatment is a full manicure plus a Bioelements cream therapy mask. Hands are soaked in warm rose-petal water enhanced with rose oil. Then the hands and lower arms are slathered with a moisturizing mask containing sesame, rosemary and peppermint oils that the skin sucks in while wrapped in cling film and heated towels. Next comes a hand massage, nail shaping, cuticle grooming and your pick of polish. By then, those hands are primed for pointing out oodles of historical landmarks.

SERVICE

Chat the afternoon away with hometown girl Gena as she fills you in on local folklore while buffing.

BOTTOM LINE

Yvette Shirey left a high-flying career as a publishing executive for the life of a small-town spa owner. "I used to frequent spas and never quite found a place that was comfortable and warm, where the people were friendly, that wasn't too uppity," she says, adding that she thought, "I can do this. I'll do it differently and make it the type of place I'd want to go — kind of like *Cheers*." And she's done just that. The locals come by for treatments, and just to chat. They sip tea and linger perhaps longer than they should. Imagine going to a spa where everybody knows your name.

INFORMATION

Golden Orchid Spa & Shop. 313 East Church Street, Frederick, MD.
Phone: (301) 695-5558. Web: http://www.goldenorchidspa.com.
The Golden Orchid signature manicure lasts one hour and costs US$40.

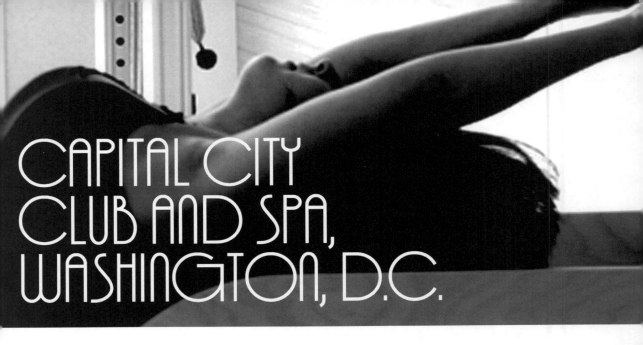

CAPITAL CITY CLUB AND SPA, WASHINGTON, D.C.

Capitol Hill is where campaigns for bills are won and lost, decisions are made to raise interest rates or increase health-care spending, and hearings are held over Watergate scandals and indiscretions with amorous interns. Talk about stressful. Good thing the Capital City Club and Spa at the Capital Hilton is open for noon spinning classes and made-for-Washington spa services such as Congressional Body Wellness and Capital Preservation Facials.

LOCATION

Much of the best of Washington is within walking distance of the hotel: the Smithsonian Institution and the White House are just three blocks away, while the Capitol building, Holocaust Museum and Washington Monument are just a short hop farther. Hip Georgetown, meanwhile, is just a short cab or subway ride removed, as are Washington Harbor, Arlington Cemetery and the Pentagon.

DESIGN

The health club and spa underwent a multimillion-dollar renovation a couple of years ago, and they look nice, but not gorgeous. Workout areas are large and stacked with weights and cardio equipment, while locker rooms are also spacious. The spa has five treatment rooms but no relaxation area, which is awkward. However, there are cushy chairs on the flipside of the locker room door, and a staffer is usually there to meet you.

CLIENTELE

Capitol Hill workers and business travellers staying at the Hilton frequent the sports club. Many take lunchtime spinning classes with Joanna or body pump with Eric — and then a Buff 'n' Bronze spa service when nobody's looking.

TREATMENTS

Reiki is a Japanese healing art that is meant to restore mental, physical and emotional balance though the light touch of healing hands. Rei means "universal," and Ki means "life force." The International Center for Reiki Training explains that "life force energy" runs through us all and is connected to our health.

Reiki is a healing technique used for stress reduction and relaxation; the "life force" is responsive to thoughts and feelings, so negative energy can cause disruptions in its flow, thereby affecting the activity of cells and organs. Reiki raises the vibratory level of the energy field in and around the body where the negative thoughts and feelings are attached, causing the negative energy to break apart and fall away, thus enabling the life force to flow in a healthy way. Sure, it may sound like a bunch of malarkey, but here's the thing: this writer went into her reiki treatment at Capitol Hill knowing zero about it and emerged a believer.

It begins with Sarah quietly introducing herself in a dimly lit room filled with the music of Enya. You lie down on a massage table and Sarah hovers her hands over your head, body and face, under the neck, then over the knees, ankles, arms and feet. She says if you can't relax, the treatment won't work. So relax. When you're finished, she will ask if you felt anything (other than supremely relaxed). You are then forced to put long-held beliefs aside and admit that some areas of your body became inexplicably hot, and that you also felt a slight vibration in your right hand. It would seem a massage doesn't necessarily have to involve deep-tissue manipulation.

Moving on to the National Relief Facial, the spa uses two different high-end skin care lines, including Dr. Grandel from Germany, which Hannah chose for my visage's combination skin. Every facial is custom made — you may be in need of extractions, two masks instead of one, a special serum, or eye cream. But it starts with a skin analysis, and includes cleansing, exfoliation, creams and a masque to seal in all those nutrients. You leave with the dewy complexion you knew you were always meant to have.

SERVICE

Sarah is sweet and soothing, and Hannah is so knowledgeable that she could write a book on skin care.

BOTTOM LINE

Whether they're here for a boot-camp class or a steam, a customized facial or Pilates, after a solid workout or a reiki treatment it would be nearly impossible to head back to Capitol Hill and be productive for the rest of the day. Which, come to think of it, isn't necessarily a bad thing.

INFORMATION

Capital City Club and Spa at the Capital Hilton. 1101 16th Street NW, Washington, D.C.. Phone: (202) 639-4300. Web: http://www.capitalcityclubandspa.com.
A half-hour reiki massage is US$55; the National Relief Facial lasts 60 minutes and costs $90.

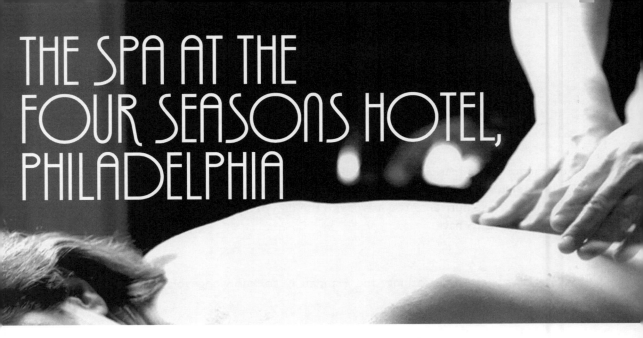

THE SPA AT THE FOUR SEASONS HOTEL, PHILADELPHIA

When you think of Philadelphia, you likely envision the Liberty Bell, Betsy Ross's house and those grease-oozing Philly cheesesteaks. That's all well and good, but I picture its vibrant arts scene, which is evident everywhere, from a mentoring and arts program that turned a 1980s graffiti problem into 2,200 downtown murals, to its pioneering efforts in funding public art that means Philly now has more of it than any other American city. In addition to the love of the arts and the brotherly love, thanks to the spa at the Four Seasons Hotel — which was just voted the best urban spa in the U.S. by *Condé Nast Traveler* readers — you can also indulge in a little love of yourself via a decadent signature spa treatment.

LOCATION

The hotel is central to the tree-lined Benjamin Franklin Parkway, a Parisian-flavoured boulevard that has become a de facto Museum Row. There's the Philadelphia Museum of Art, the Rodin Museum, the Franklin Institute, Moore College of Art, the Please Touch Museum for Children and the Academy of Natural Sciences, to name a few. There are "Walk Philadelphia" signs with clear instructions on just about every major street corner, so you know that the majestic City Hall is only a five-minute stroll from the hotel, the ritzy Rittenhouse Square is a meandering ten, and the Reading Terminal Market — where Philly has been filling up for more than a century on everything from Amish baked goods to soul food and homemade ice cream — is fifteen. As an added bonus, when you're on your walkabout you'll see the widest variety of urban architecture to be found in the United States.

DESIGN

The Four Seasons may look smallish from the outside, but within you'll find a large and lovely hotel of 364 rooms and suites that boast a contemporary flair fused with Philly-appropriate Federal-style furniture. The lobby level is extremely welcoming, with its rose-tinted marble, oversized seating areas, antiques and deluxe floral arrangements. The spa and fitness facility, with its gym, sauna and steam rooms, are intimate and cozy, home to nature sounds, marble-topped counters and cloth wall-paper in muted tones. On the way through the fitness area towards the change room, cranberry water, Gatorade, apples and tea are all available. The handful of treatment rooms feature wall sconces and stylish throws on massage beds. Best is the pool area, which is like a little tropical oasis of mirrors and ferns, terry cloth–lined chaise longues, a massive whirlpool, a blue lap pool and a few bistro tables and chairs for spa alternative cuisine. By night, balconies and windows garner magical views of the elegant museum facades done up in dramatic lighting.

CLIENTELE

The regular Four Seasons socialites and business people who are willing to pay US$400 a night for all of those elegant extras.

TREATMENTS

Facials include the Four Seasons Liberty and Skin Renewal, while body treatments feature Lemon Water Ice Exfoliation and the Four Seasons in One experience. Their signature massage is the Philadelphia Freedom Hot Towel Infusion. It goes like this: Heather, who is dressed almost like a hospital orderly in green scrubs (they take this stuff seriously), has you sniff a special herbal elixir that has been positioned below the face cradle. This is meant to open up the senses and mind and prepare the body for the massage and a lashing of hot towels steeped and steamed in a lavender-and-geranium infusion. The hot, wet terry towels are pushed into the muscle areas (ahhh), warming them up for a Swedish massage, which is administered with gusto — not to mention 100 percent plant-based oils. The hot towel and massage steps are then repeated, yielding double the pleasure.

FOOD & DRINK

Logan Square, one of the five public spaces in William Penn's original plan for the city of Philadelphia, boasts the Fountain of the Three Rivers, an ornate watery feature and the namesake of the Four Seasons' Fountain Restaurant, home of the best jacket-required dinners in the city. Chef Martin Hamann offers up fresh market cuisine such as American foie gras with quince ravioli dressed with a cider vinegar sauce, and grilled rabbit tenderloin with a terrine of rabbit confit, caramelized apples and toasted walnut sauce. Healthier, nutritionally balanced fare is available from the restaurants and from room service. And if you're looking for a lively post-spa cocktail hour, check out the restaurant's abutting Swann Lounge. *Gourmet* magazine has rated Fountain Philadelphia's top table, and lauds the Swann Lounge as the top hotel bar worldwide.

SERVICE

The J-Lo vehicle *Maid in Manhattan* was filmed here, and if you saw that flick you no doubt learned that it takes an army of managers, housekeepers, concierges, doormen, valets, waiters and spa workers to dish out that famous Four Seasons service. Think in-room exercise equipment, top-notch aestheticians, non-allergenic pillows, bedtime milk and cookies for the kiddies and, for Rover, fresh-baked dog biscuits and Evian in a silver bowl.

BOTTOM LINE

The spa may be small, but it's an immensely popular and enjoyable experience in the heart of a city that's full of heart.

INFORMATION

Four Seasons Hotel Philadelphia. One Logan Square (North 18th Street at Benjamin Franklin Parkway), Philadelphia, PA.
Phone: (215) 405-2815. Web: http://www.fourseasons.com/philadelphia. The Philadelphia Freedom Hot Towel Infusion Ultimate Experience lasts 80 minutes and costs US$175.

SPATOPIA

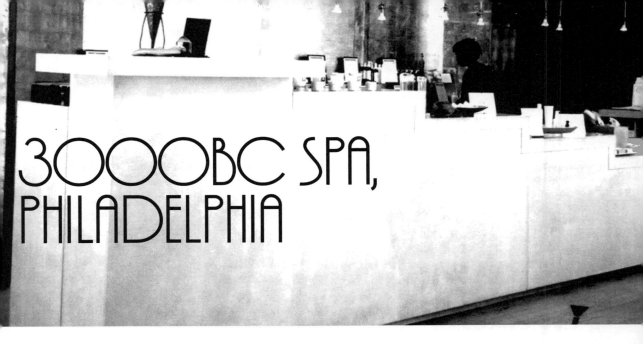

3OOOBC SPA, PHILADELPHIA

Drive out of downtown Philadelphia — or any major city centre in the United States, for that matter — and you never know what you'll find. Perhaps there's nothing but abandoned railway tracks or a rundown truck stop. Or you could discover a pristine garden district such as Chestnut Hill, where the *crème de la crème* of Philly society resides in centuries-old stone homes tucked away off a cobblestone thoroughfare. On this same street you'll find 3000BC, one of the first aromatherapy spas on the East Coast and one that Philadelphians are just now discovering a dozen years after it opened. In 2001, it was voted Best Holistic Spa in the annual Best of Philly survey. It also won Best Facials and Best Body Treatments honours in 2002.

Photo by Amy Rosen

LOCATION

The spa is on Germantown Avenue, the main strip of Chestnut Hill, a community where the air smells of fresh rain, lilac and everything else you would expect in faux small-town Philly. It is flanked by CinCin, an upscale Chinese-French fusion eatery; the Solaris Grille, which serves an award-winning chopped salad; the deck at the charming Chestnut Hill Hotel; and, for the best in unnecessary knick-knacks, boutiques such as the Little Nook, Kitchen Kapers, Yankee Candle Company and Simple Cottage.

DESIGN

For a decade, 3000BC was tucked away in the back of a grand Dutch colonial building, where an antique store occupied most of the space. But as of the summer of 2003, the antique vendors had recently closed up shop and the spa embarked on plans to take over the entire first floor, adding four treatment rooms, a locker and shower facility, and manicure and pedicure stations. At the time of writing, there were three treatment rooms around the back and down the stairs.

The spa space is raw and minimalist, but it's neither Zen oasis nor Holly Hobby feminine. It's more of an austere environment, with white walls and industrial grey carpeting. It's what a spa would look like if you and your best friend were to decide to convert your basement into a holistic rumpus room.

The 3000BC Boutique — a holistic corner store that actually predates the spa — is an attractive open space with high ceilings, large windows and gleaming gold-leaf walls. Items for sale include its own line of aromatherapy oils and lotions, salts and skin care products. To properly re-create your favourite treatments at home, buy the products along with the specific "environment" CD engineered to go along with various spa services. There's one for aromatherapy, reflexology and *reiki*, among others. This is New Age music that actually adds to a treatment instead of acting as an annoying distraction.

CLIENTELE

Affluent Chestnut Hill residents have been the spa's core clientele, but in recent years positive press has brought in other suburbanites. And because of the gender-free environs, men make up a good portion of the spa's visitors.

TREATMENTS

Most body treatments are organic and holistic, while the skin care services, such as resurfacing glycolic peels and revitalizing eye treatments, bridge the gap between holistic and scientific methods.

Aromatherapy facial with microdermabrasion spot treatments, anyone? Other spa specialties include such well-being services as craniosacral therapy, hypnotherapy and shiatsu. Try their Philly survey–winning Saqqara Body Treatment, which uses a grainy, fragrant mix of jojoba beads and sunflower, lemon and almond oils, followed by a firming body infusion oil that contains juniper, lemon and lavender. The end result is meant to improve circulation and reduce cellulite. It's a very relaxing, methodical treatment — wax on, wax off — with no surprises. The firming body infusion helps tighten and tone the skin, while the saqqara polish sloughs off errant dead cells.

Hot terry towels are used to wash away both concoctions, and then a moisturizing lotion brings you back to your original lustre. All the while, you receive a Swedish massage coupled with a bit of pressure on any notable tight spots. It's both relaxing and rejuvenating, and you know the treatment has worked its magic when you emerge feeling both woozy and energized.

SERVICE

The young, skilled staff are all decked out in black 3000BC T-shirts. Massage therapist Lilla has that winning combination of soft voice and strong hands.

BOTTOM LINE

3000BC is an anti-fabulous spot where it's not about who's who and what they're wearing in decadent day spa surroundings. It's a laid-back neighbourhood haunt where the emphasis is on therapy, training and the products they use. And then, feasting upon homemade ice cream while candle-shopping the afternoon away.

INFORMATION

3000BC Spa and Boutique. 7946 Germantown Avenue, Philadelphia, PA.
Phone: (215) 247-6020 or 1-800-AROMATIC (1-800-276-6284).
Web: http://www.3000bc.com.
The hour-long Aromatherapy Body Polish and Firming Body Infusion costs US$95.

SPATOPIA

ELIZABETH ARDEN RED DOOR SALON & SPA, NEW YORK

There's something to be said for consumer insight: knowing what the public wants, conceiving of a related product or service, then dispensing it in winning style. Take spas, for example: as recently as twenty years ago, most North Americans thought of them as places to go for manicures or to "recuperate" from "minor facial surgery" in "Switzerland." Now you can't fling a jar of eucalyptus salt scrub in a high-end shopping district without hitting a masseuse in the head.

The more the merrier, but let's give credit where it's due: at almost a century old, Elizabeth Arden Red Door Salons & Spas were pampering pusses long before customized phyto-organic facials with olive oil lip treatments were even a twinkle in our contour-creamed eyes. With twenty-seven Red Doors throughout the United States and Europe, they remain the industry leader.

LOCATION

Eleven Red Doors are placed in Marshall Field's and Saks Fifth Avenue stores across the country, including this New York outpost on Fifth Avenue. When day spa meets power shopping, can it be anything but a dream team? Located on the concourse level of Saks, the dedicated Red Door elevator takes you from the bowels of Bobbi Brown, Burberry, DKNY and D&G up to four floors and 30,000 square feet of retail, hair and nail, skin care and body services.

If shopping's not your speed, go for a skate at neighbouring Rockefeller Center, or cross the street and grab a gourmet java and a lemon square at Dean & DeLuca. Then put on your goofiest grin and wave to Katie and Matt through the *Today* show windows across the plaza.

DESIGN

Walk through the eponymous red door and into the ground floor makeup and skin product boutique with its splashy crimson walls. Up in the spa area you'll find a contrary colour scheme of muted greens, ecru and burnished silver, which is fine. But the layout and the aggressively efficient use of space are a sticking point: the last thing you want when you visit a spa is to feel like a piece of veal; but that's precisely the image conjured up by the row of curtained pens (a.k.a. cubicles) where you change from street gear into spa gear (hand off the bag for your shoes and hanger for your clothes to an attendant). There is a relaxation area stocked with teas, water and a big bowl of Japanese cracker mix, but nobody's sitting there. There's no time.

CLIENTELE

It's all about high volume and getting things done in a New York minute. You'll notice scores of stressed-out men and women checking in at the exact same moment as you, and you'll encounter them again (albeit looking infinitely more relaxed) in precisely fifty minutes. No dawdling or dilly-dallying. Get your massage, leave the knots behind and hit the road.

TREATMENTS

Let's face it: life is exhausting. Especially during sale seasons, what with all that bending and buttoning, pulling and lacing, wrestling and hair-pulling... Red Door's new Elemental Balancing Massage is a good fit. It features fragrant blends of essential oils created to meet your personal healing objectives. The Balancing Blend is meant to relieve sore and tired muscles, calm and soothe the nerves; Detoxifying Blend is for cellulite and water retention; Stress-Relieving Blend is, logically enough, there for relaxation and tension reduction; Loving Blend may aid in self-nurturing, balancing and strengthening, plus it opens the heart to joy; Revitalizing Blend is for energizing, uplifting, stimulating and refreshing. If only you could choose them all.

Once you've selected your mood blend, a combination of advanced hands-on massage techniques is used on the body, including Swedish, Acupressure, Lymph Drainage and Reflexology. Victoria gives a masterful rubdown that is relentlessly relaxing, while the chosen aromatic blends reduce stress, detoxify and sure do smell pretty. An added benefit is that the oils stimulate the olfactory centres of the brain, creating different physiological effects to enhance beauty, health and well-being. So while you may look good, you'll feel fabulous.

Other treatments range from breast surgery massage, green tea manicures and photography makeup application to back waxing and a phyto-organic anti-cellulite leg treatment with take-home program.

SERVICE

Pleasant and polished with that patented New York hustle.

BOTTOM LINE

You don't stick around in the beauty biz for a century by simply batting your eyelashes and looking pretty. This is a well-oiled engine that'll likely keep chugging into the next century, but one hopes the Red Doors don't forget that they're in the business of wellness and relaxation. And that means leaving time to stop and smell the essential oil blends every once in a while.

INFORMATION

Elizabeth Arden Red Door Salon & Spa. 611 Fifth Avenue at 50th Street, New York, NY.
Phone: (212) 940-4000. You can book appointments for any of their spas online at http://www.reddoorsalons.com. The Elemental Balancing Massage lasts 50 minutes and costs US$95.

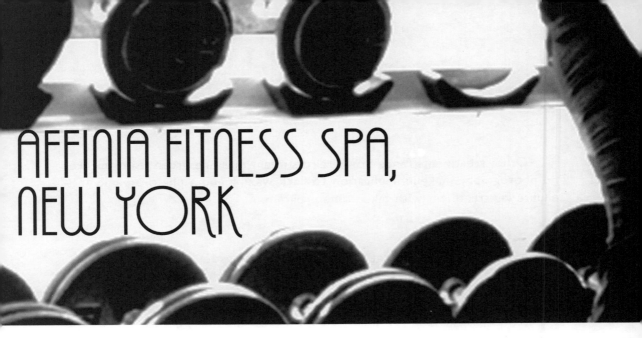

AFFINIA FITNESS SPA, NEW YORK

Bad news, lazy bones. Next time you go to New York City, you'll have no excuse for skipping your regular workout now that the newly rebranded Affinia Fitness Spa at the Affinia Dumont has opened.

After a US$15 million renovation, Manhattan's first (and so far only) fitness suite hotel has re-emerged as an "it" spot for the health-conscious business traveller. For starters, there's a fitness concierge on staff who arranges appointments with personal trainers, leads yoga classes in the lobby and has free loaner Fit Kits sent to your room (to help with running or strength training). The mini-bar is full of healthy treats — energy bars and low-fat snacks. They've even got "black books" of NYC fitness resources, restaurants with healthy food options, runners' maps (and towels and a water bottle upon your return) and, of course, the spa itself.

With treatments like the Fat Burner and the Sport Pack, it's finally happened: fitness club has met spa.

LOCATION

The Murray Hill neighbourhood in the heart of midtown Manhattan is an historic enclave that's near all the essentials. You can walk down the street to Madison Avenue and its shops, or Seventh Avenue and *its* shops. Macy's, one of the world's largest department stores, is also a hop, skip and a credit-card advance away. And after you've finished shopping, Madison Square Garden, Times Square, Penn Station and the Empire State Building are all nearby.

DESIGN

The spa includes the small, bright, glassed-in fitness centre, seven treatment rooms, large locker areas and a relaxation room. Earth tones permeate throughout, but are boosted by blond wood and colourful graphic carpeting. In other words, it's got that modern boutique-hotel vibe.

CLIENTELE

Mostly health-minded professionals looking for a little balance in their workaday lives. A good portion are business travellers, but some are fitness club members (who get 10 percent off all treatments) and increasingly the spa-goers are men. "They come here and figure, 'Strange town, why not give it a try? My buddies won't see me,'" says therapist Caitlin, who has given many hotel guests their first-ever Men's Conditioning Facial.

SPATOPIA

TREATMENTS

The philosophy of the spa is that everyone needs balance in their lives, and that includes maintaining a continuous level of fitness and restoring the body's natural balance. For the former, there's the Life Fitness treadmills, Total Body Crosstrainers, Upright Lifecycles, personal trainers and all the weight-training apparatus in the gym. For the latter, there are facials and body treatments, massage therapies and grooming services. All use the Avance line of skin care products that utilize the curative properties of natural elements such as seaweed from the Brittany coast of France.

Many services bridge the gap between superficial and therapeutic, and the therapists recommend incorporating exercise into your spa experience. "A cellulite treatment alone isn't going to get rid of cellulite," Caitlin explains. "Sure, it'll increase circulation and even things out, but exercise is needed for more extensive results."

For those who've gone overboard with the exercise, treatments include the seaweed-wrap Decompression Zone and the Muscular Ease Body Dip, during which your entire body is wrapped in a blanket of warm paraffin.

To ease forehead pressure and allergies from the changing seasons and to purify the skin, the Sinus Relief Facial is just what the doctor ordered. It starts with a skin analysis, followed by cleansing, toning, exfoliating, and deep steam inhalation boosted by an energizing remedy — an essential-oil blend containing peppermint and eucalyptus. Then Caitlin uses pressure-point stimulation techniques on the sinus areas, offers up hand and scalp massages, and lays on the purifying cream, a mask and a vitamin C amulet to rev up the regeneration of cells and calm inflammation and puffiness.

It's a whole bag of tricks for the face, and you leave looking good and breathing a little easier.

SERVICE

Imagine having someone restore your sense of smell by giving you a facial. Who knew?

BOTTOM LINE

Is it a hotel or a health club? A spa or a spot for lifestyle makeovers? Perhaps all of the above. And instead of putting on a few pounds the next time you go to NYC on a business trip, you might end up getting in shape.

INFORMATION

Affinia Fitness Spa at the Affinia Dumont. 150 East 34th Street, New York, NY. Phone: (212) 545-5254. Web: http://www.affinia.com.
The Sinus Relief facial lasts about an hour and costs US$90. The fitness centre is free for hotel guests; monthly or annual local memberships are also available. A full year costs $850.

AVON SALON AND SPA, NEW YORK

They call it the "five-minute facelift," and short of signing up for TV's *Extreme Makeover*, nothing can change a person's look more — or more instantly — than a good eyebrow shaping.

Eliza Petrescu has been the chief waxing director and eyebrow designer at Avon Salon & Spa since it opened in 1998, and she is also the namesake and visionary behind its first boutique dedicated to the art of eyebrow shaping: Eliza's Eyes @ Avon Salon & Spa.

Famous for pioneering the classically elongated eyebrow shape, Petrescu has transformed the brow into an extension of haute couture. With one long, steady gaze, she (or her highly trained roster of associates) intuitively knows what is needed to sculpt perfect eyebrows.

Which is why I'm here.

Not long ago, I was sitting at a bar when a leggy model plunked down beside me, introduced herself, then looked me in the eyes and said, "You'd be so much prettier if you did something about those brows."

When intoxicated strangers start offering up spontaneous personal grooming tips, you should probably listen. And take action. Because, just like children, they often speak the truth.

LOCATION

The Avon Salon & Spa takes up three floors in the gilded Trump Tower on Fifth Avenue, smack-dab in the middle of perhaps the most perfect shopping street in the universe. The first floor is dedicated to retail; Eliza's Eyes is on the second; and the spa treatment rooms are on the sixth.

DESIGN

The retail shop is glossed-up white marble. Up the spiral staircase, you come upon a row of sandblasted glass pods with white curtains, where cushy dentist-style chairs and specialty lighting encourage perfect arches. The rest of the floor is all wood and chrome, and walls decked with framed write-ups about Petrescu from magazines such as *Allure*, *New York* and *O*. Up on the sixth floor, the modern aesthetic of the rest of the spa gives way to a nineteenth-century parlour vibe, including goldenrod carpets, textured wallpaper and mahogany furnishings.

CLIENTELE

Not only is the second floor packed with New York urbanites waiting for their fifteen-minute refreshers, but the rich and famous also fly in from around the globe to get plucked by the "Queen of the Arch." Petrescu has done everyone from Halle Berry and J. Lo to Natasha Richardson and Jennifer Grey, who declares in the brochure that "Eliza gives me the eyebrows that I'm sure God meant me to have."

TREATMENTS

The sixth floor provides fine French pedicures and cellulite-busting Endermologie treatments; hot stone, pre- and postnatal massages; hair and makeup services; and even personal Hatha yoga sessions. But the staff on the second floor are here for one thing and one thing only: beautiful brows.

They call your name from the long list of those awaiting their power-plucking session, then you glide into a glass pod, ease into the reclining chair, and are covered with a smock. A high-beam magnifying glass shines over your face, then Petrescu or an associate hands you a mirror and, using the thin handle of a small eyebrow brush, they illustrate what they plan to do.

Now, I've long considered my magic-marker-like eyebrows a bit of a trademark; I keep them groomed, but I've never had them professionally shaped. "Yes, I can tell," offers the helpful associate. "I'll show you what is wrong. They're too round; you plucked too much underneath. See, here you tried to make an arch. This is not the way to make an arch. The arch is over here. Not here.

"I'm going to take a bit away from here to make them more even. Some places I can take, some places you can grow. On the top we have to follow the same line. I'm going to even out the top."

She says the shaping rules follow the eye. To determine the proper brow shape and length, there's a lesson involving the nose and inside corner of the eye, outer edge of the iris, nostrils and temples. The eyebrows also grow according to the shape of the bones.

Another thing to take into account is the shape of the face: "That's why we don't do the same eyebrows for everyone." After about fifteen minutes of tweezing, waxing and snipping, I'm done. But there's homework: "You still have a little place here you have to grow before I can give you your perfect arch."

BOTTOM LINE

Do not attempt a big brow change on your own. Sure, you can clean up a bit to look presentable, but it's best to leave the shaping process to the professionals. Eyebrows are a homegrown accessory that can make or break a face, and this is a spa treatment that reveals total improvement in ten to fifteen minutes. Mine turned out to be pretty much what I started with, albeit a sleeker, more defined and overall better-looking version of the originals. All in all, I think the drunken model would be duly impressed.

INFORMATION

Avon Salon & Spa. 725 Fifth Avenue (between 56th and 57th streets), New York, NY Phone: (212) 755-2866. Web: http://www.avonsalonandspa.com. An initial visit with Eliza Petrescu costs US$100. "Maintenance" visits run $78. A session with one of Petrescu's associates is $45.

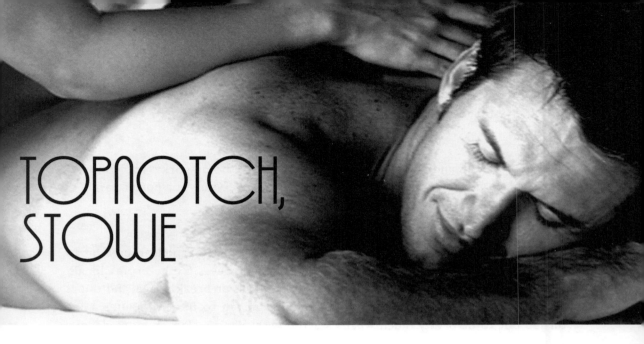

TOPNOTCH, STOWE

*S*towe is a little nugget of a town where each of the four seasons plays a crucial role in attracting outdoorsy tourists for leaf peeping, pristine winter skiing, and perhaps best of all, springtime hikes along wildflower-dotted paths. Not one to let nature's fragrant bounty go to waste, the spa at Topnotch uses such New England favourites as maple sugar and local herbs and wildflowers in its body wraps, polishes and scrubs. When the hills come alive with lavender and violets, so does the spa.

LOCATION

Vermont's lush Green Mountains provide the majestic backdrop for Topnotch, and the surrounding rivers, hills and dales offer world-renowned biking and skiing, hiking atop Mount Mansfield, excellent canoeing, fly fishing, tennis and two scoops at the legendary Ben and Jerry's ice cream factory.

DESIGN

Topnotch is located on a fifty-hectare wooded estate at the foot of Mount Mansfield, about eight kilometres from the village of Stowe. The lobby area has that perfect ski-lodge vibe, complete with focal-point fireplace and looming giant moose head. The resort has 110 rooms and 12 suites dressed up with antiques and designer flourishes, all of which are spacious and welcoming. The two- and three-bedroom townhouses — which are family favourites — have fireplaces, saunas, whirlpools and sundecks. The 2,000-square-metre spa features woodsy interiors, lots of natural stonework and walls of glass, which yield panoramic mountain views. The massive indoor pool and equally impressive whirlpool add to their *ahhh* factor with cascading hydromassage waterfalls. Along with the Tennis Academy, cardio studios and a fitness schedule that goes from strength to strength via offerings like Belly Dance, Chinese Yoga, Sports Training Circuit and Aqua Aerobics, Topnotch definitely lives up to its billing as a luxury resort. And even though the spa may be looking a little worse for wear, it's in the midst of an extensive renovation to expand and beautify.

CLIENTELE

The resort appeals to such a cross-section of society; you've got your granola types, loads of men, families, amorous couples and, as always, gaggles of women on getaway weekends.

TREATMENTS

More than ninety different treatments are up for grabs, from aroma mountain massages and Vermont river rock treatments to manual dermabrasion and even a shampoo and set. The two most popular are the maple sugar scrub and the Vermont wildflower treatment. For the latter, Amy guides you into the first room, all wet white tiles, for a loofah scrub with sea salt and lavender soap. Then she hoses you down. Up you get, pad down the hall and enter another room, where you lie down on another massage table and are wrapped in linen sheets that have been steeped in a hot tea of wildflowers and herbs such as spearmint (soothes nerves, calms, tones and purifies), comfrey root (tightens skin and regenerates), thyme (cleanses and purifies), violets (balances) and roses (softens and moisturizes). You lie there sweating and detoxifying, then trot along to a final room for a Swedish massage, kicked up with wildflower oil. Local herbalist Louise Downey has created these natural blends especially for Topnotch. At the end of this triple-threat treatment, you receive a take-home bag of loofah, lavender soap and the most delicious Vermont maple sugar hard candies you'll ever taste.

A couple of years ago, the spa began offering its maple sugar body scrub as a gentler alternative to traditional salt-based scrubs. The yummy maple sugar is supplied by a nearby farm, and the scrub is enriched with vegetable oils, antioxidants and a handful of vitamins. Afterwards, you'll feel as soft as a kitten, and the great taste will leave you licking your paws.

FOOD & DRINK

There's morning coffee in the living room, summertime poolside lunches at the Gazebo, and the Buttertub Bistro for drinks, pub fare and live music. Maxwell's is the elegant dining room both for gourmet spa cuisine (healthy choices list their calorie and fat counts on the menu) as well as innovative market-influenced dishes such as herb-crusted rack of lamb with polenta and grilled vegetables, or smoked salmon on blini, sauced with lemon beurre blanc. Maxwell's comprehensive wine list has received *Wine Spectator*'s award of excellence and is one of the finest collections in the region.

SERVICE

Perhaps a wee bit matter-of-fact, but they get the job done with aplomb.

BOTTOM LINE

If all of the nature, exercise and relaxation and wildflowers weren't enough, there's always Ben and Jerry's on the ride home.

INFORMATION

Topnotch. 4000 Mountain Road, Stowe, VT. Phone: 1-800-451-8686 or (802) 253-8585. Web: http://www.topnotch-resort.com.
Rooms start at US$175 per night. The Vermont Wildflower Treatment lasts 80 minutes and costs $150. The Maple Sugar Body Scrub lasts 25 minutes and costs $60.

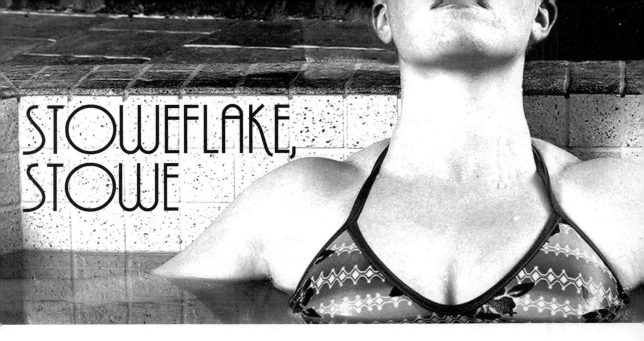

STOWEFLAKE, STOWE

Well-groomed ladies cornered the spa market more than a decade ago, long before the new millennium ushered in the rise of the pampered male. Now seniors are one of the fastest-growing spa demographics, and even teenage girls have their own people proffering group pedicures and acne-clearing facials. So, we've covered all the bases, right? Teens, some tweens, and men and women of all ages. But not so fast — what about the children?

Stoweflake Mountain Resort & Spa became an industry trailblazer by launching a new Kids' Spa Menu. That's right — real spa treatments for real kids (aged seven and up). Goodbye natural exfoliation via the backyard sandbox; hello to the US$100 Mini-Maple body scrub.

LOCATION

Stowe is a charming, kid-friendly tourist town nestled amidst Vermont's lush Green Mountains. Stoweflake is a forty-five-minute drive from Burlington, Vermont, and about two and a half hours from Montreal. Historic Stowe Village is home to such shops as Mountain Sport and Bikes, Stowe Maple Products and, for anglers, the Fly Rod Shop & Fly Fish Vermont. The Stowe Recreation Path cuts a swath through it all. Oh, and the Ben and Jerry's ice cream factory is just down the road.

DESIGN

The overall look of Stoweflake, one of New England's only resorts to earn a Four Diamond rating from AAA, is warm without being country. There are wooden pillars, curved glass and natural stone. Cork covers the treatment room floors, and there's a courtyard with a rustic covered bridge and herbal and meditation gardens. There are restaurants, shops, boardrooms and ballrooms, as well as 137 guest rooms and suites, including eleven Spa Suites located just above the new spa expansion.

The spa and fitness area encompasses 50,000 square feet with thirty treatment rooms, men's and women's private sanctuaries, separate kids' spa rooms in the older fitness wing, several saunas and steam rooms, a sunken Jacuzzi, solarium, spa café, massive yoga and fitness studios, dedicated spinning room, indoor and outdoor swimming pools (open year-round; the kids love it), private consultation rooms (for lifestyle counselling in nutrition, fitness and even physiotherapy), the spa gift shop and salon.

A focal point is the unisex aqua solarium, a manmade grotto with mountain views. The Bingham Falls Hot Springs Hydrotherapy — inspired by the local falls

— is a thunderous four-metre-high water feature designed to massage back, neck and shoulders at a temperature of 36 degrees Celsius. While modern, the spa incorporates the outdoor beauty of Vermont.

CLIENTELE

Kids running around every which way, amorous couples, conventioneers, après-skiers in tuques, and gaggles of women on spa getaways. In short, anyone and everyone. In fact, spa director Chris Pulito says Stoweflake has invented a new category: resort destination spa. "You can do just about anything — take a Nordic walking snowshoe class, go for a sleigh ride with the kids, come here for total spa immersion and then go to the dining room for filet mignon with bordelaise sauce. Or, come for a week for foliage, yoga classes, a maple syrup scrub and have spa cuisine delivered to your suite."

TREATMENTS

There are more than 120 treatments to choose from, many of which celebrate the local seasons and indigenous ingredients such as wildflowers and wood spice. The Stowe Après-Ski Massage — which is just as good after a Pilates class — is Swedish, with some stretching and pressure-point techniques, heat therapy and oils. The kicker is that your hands and feet are wrapped in hot, moist towels, perfect for getting the blood circulating in those frostbitten toes.

The Kids Spa Menu is full of sugar and spice and everything nice. For now, there are six treatments: Kids Massage, Massage Sampler, Aroma Massage, Mini-Massage, Rose Bud Wrap and Mini-Maple. They all last forty-five minutes, except for the Mini-Massage, which lasts twenty. The descriptions of the treatments are the same as their adult counterparts, but Pulito says a gentler touch is used. The children's treatment rooms are separate from the main spa (which they are not allowed to enter), and a guardian must be in the room at all times during treatments. The children must wear bathing suits. So far, Pulito says, the Kids Menu has been a smashing success.

FOOD & DRINK

Even though it's a so-called pub, Charlie B's has its food prepared by the same four-diamond chef as the resort's fine-dining restaurant, and it also happens to be a *Wine Spectator* magazine award winner, offering fifty wines by the glass in a casual, ski-lodge atmosphere. Menu choices run the gamut from yakitori beef short ribs to Buffalo-style rock shrimp with chunky blue cheese dressing, and even a daily fish offering. I ordered a spa bento box that included a mini-bowl of deeply flavoured onion soup (sans crust of cheese), Bibb lettuce salad with hazelnut dressing, moist poached salmon on a black bean, corn and avocado succotash, and a piece of some-how decadent yet dairy-free cheesecake with blueberry compote. The kids' menu comes with crayons, riddles and appetizers such as creamy clam chowder, as well as mains like burgers and home-style macaroni and cheese.

Winfield's Bistro offers more upscale service and menu options. Choices include beef carpaccio with remulata, fleur de sel and petite greens; and braised lamb shank with winter vegetable ragout and horseradish potato mousse.

SERVICE

New England warm without being too homey. The spa attendants wear polo shirts and khakis, and are ever present and helpful.

BOTTOM LINE

Are these new children's treatments a disturbing money grab, or a visionary trend whose time has come? After all, kids play harder than most of us, so presumably they could benefit from massage. And learning to take care of their bodies at a young age can't be a bad thing. Even so, the idea makes me a little uncomfortable. But I'm totally sold on Stoweflake as a resort where everyone can go away together for some great family fun.

INFORMATION

Stoweflake Mountain Resort & Spa. 1746 Mountain Road, Stowe, VT.
Phone: (802) 253-7355. Web: http://www.stoweflake.com.
Kids' spa services range from US$50 for a Mini-Massage to $100 for the Rose Bud Wrap or Mini-Maple body treatments. The Stowe Après-Ski Massage lasts 80 minutes and costs $130.

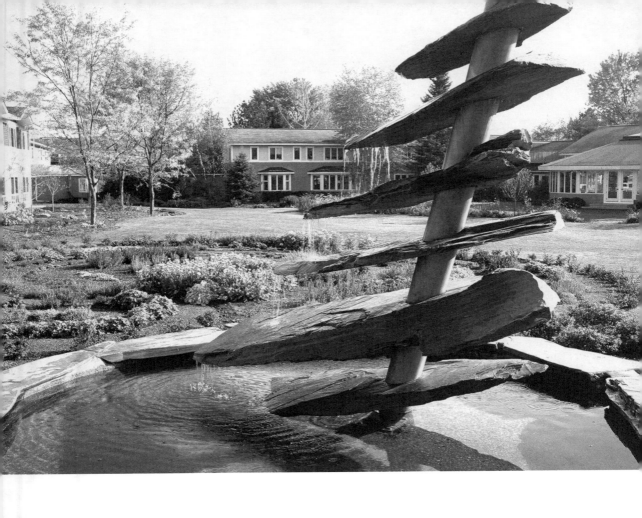

SPATOPIA

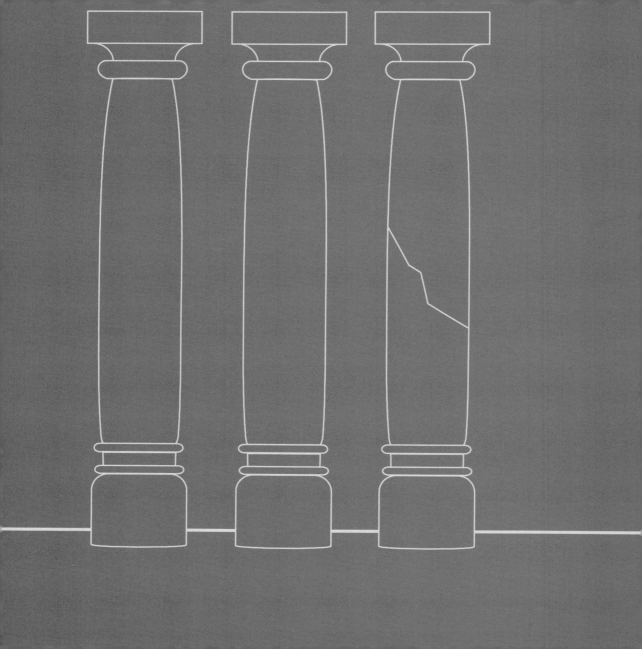

INTERNATIONAL SPAS

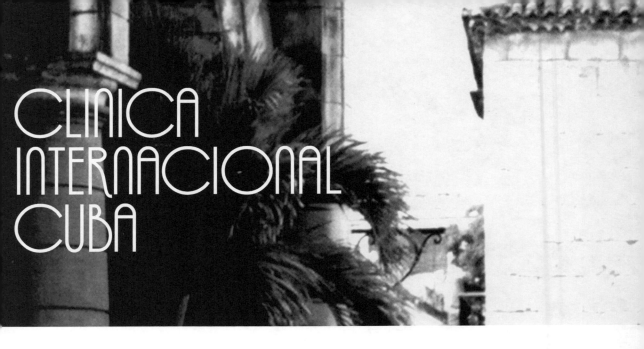

CLINICA INTERNACIONAL CUBA

Booking a spa treatment at a clinic in a communist country may not seem like the best-laid plan. But when you consider that Cuba boasts free healthcare for all who live there, getting your mud massage from a doctor trained in reflexology doesn't seem like such an aberration.

After the collapse of the Soviet Union in the 1980s, cash-strapped Cuba was forced to seek out an approach to medicine that was cheaper and more readily available. Officials soon discovered that homeopathy, Chinese medicine and naturopathy weren't only economical, but also produced excellent results. Now widely used throughout the country, the techniques have triggered a minor boom in health tourism amongst frazzled capitalists in need of some seaside stress relief.

Photo by Amy Rosen

LOCATION

Varadero is a lively little resort town located on the Hicacos Peninsula on the northern coast of Matanzas province. It's a two-hour drive along a scenic coastal highway from Cuba's capital city, Havana. The beach is just a coconut's throw away. In town, you'll find a massive crafts market brimming with woodcarvings, hand-tooled leather goods and vibrant paintings. Varadero also boasts good restaurants (featuring Alberta beef), a hot nightlife and endless aquatic activities, including scuba diving, surfing, and sailing or cruising adventures with such well-oiled outfits as Jolly Roger. The historic city of Matanzas is nearby, and one hour south is Zapata Peninsula Grand Nature Park.

Then again, you might just choose to grease up and roast on the beach beside turquoise waters with an icy mojito highball in hand.

Havana is not far off, and spending at least one day amidst its colonial architecture, spicy culture and signs of good things to come is a must. It has always had character to spare, but now Old Havana is being restored to her former glory, thanks to the Cuban Hoteliers Association and a UNESCO designation as a World Heritage Site. The place now looks like a million bucks. Have an espresso at Café Taberna, where some members of the Buena Vista Social Club play daily, then stop by one of Ernest Hemingway's favourite haunts, La Bodeguita del Medio, for a hand-rolled Cohiba.

DESIGN

Communist chic: celery-green floor tiles, sterile white walls, regulation-issue furniture, ceiling fans, framed photos of Castro and Che Guevara, doors and shutters flung open to greet the ocean breeze.

CLIENTELE

Locals, including a healthy-looking girl, an elderly woman and a middle-aged man, sit outside in the sun, waiting to be called into the physiotherapy room at the clinic. Most patients, however, are tourists from Canada, Germany, Spain and Argentina. Elderly snowbirds come for relief from arthritis (massage and such), while high-flying executives come for the anti-stress program (based on psychology, reflexology, and relaxation techniques). In this program, each session lasts about an hour and a half for a minimum of four days a week. Within a few sessions patients have noted promising results, without Western medications.

TREATMENTS

There are two distinct programs offered at the clinic: medical assistance (scooter mishaps, for example) and quality of life. Eighty percent of the patients are here for the latter (the Cuban healthcare system has its heart in preventative medicine). The first and second tiers of the quality-of-life system — massage, facials and other cosmetic treatments, although the second level includes more complex treatments like acupuncture, reflexology and mud therapies — are based at the hotels. The third takes place at the clinic: you meet with a medical team composed of a doctor, a psychologist and a chiropractor or physiotherapist. Together, they design a holistic program, tailored to remedy such problems as anxiety.

But if you had, say, problems with night cramping in your feet, you could see Nelson, a charming doctor who studied reflexology for four years at the University of Havana Medical School. Strong hands, local black mud and the necessity for a high pain threshold are all part of this reflexology massage. Nelson says his brawny technique conjures up "a grateful pain." It's true. Relaxed feet plus smooth skin equals one happy tourist. And you can pick up a tube of sunburn-relief gel made from the local plant *sabadilla* on your way out.

FOOD & DRINK

Cuba has unfairly acquired a bad rep when it comes to its native cuisine: rice and beans, fried plantains, squash, steak and potatoes, and local lobster and shrimp — all fresh, all delicious. With a meat-and-cheese Cubano sandwich on a crusty bun in one hand and a daiquiri in the other, just try to complain. Without a full mouth.

SERVICE

The people are as warm as the Cuban sun. A mustachioed doctor holds a lit cigarette behind his back as he talks animatedly through a translator. A pharmacy worker wears a '50s-style white nurse's uniform while dispensing sought-after locally made drugs such as PPG-5 (made from sugar cane and said to lower cholesterol levels). Although healthcare staff are poorly paid — doctors make a pittance — they appear satisfied with their work.

BOTTOM LINE

Communism never felt so good. Book a week-long vacation at an all-inclusive resort, take in an anti-stress program at the clinic and go home a sun-kissed, healthier, happier you.

INFORMATION

Clinica Internacional Varadero. 1st Avenue and 1st Street, Varadero, Cuba. Phone: 011-53-45-66-7710. Email: clinica@clinica.var.cyt.cu. Clinica Internacional is open 24 hours. It is part of Servimed, a health-tourism network that includes thirty members ranging from Clinica Internacional all the way up to spas in five-star resorts. Prices are very reasonable (US$20 for a two-hour massage, for example), but costs vary from clinic to hotel to resort.

SANDALS ROYAL BAHAMIAN RESORT AND SPA, BAHAMAS

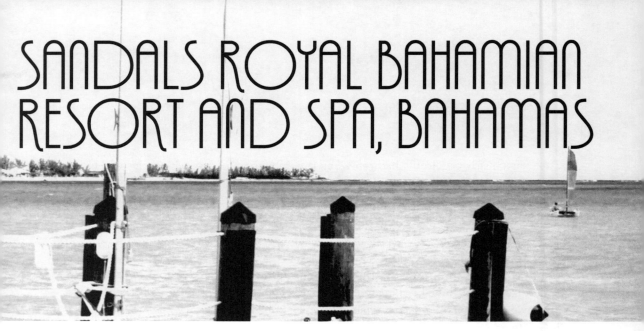

When it's cold and icy and you've had it up to here with playing charades, why not head someplace steamy for a mid-winter break, like a long weekend in the Bahamas?

It's easier than you think; just a three-hour early-morning flight from Toronto, followed by a quick jaunt from the Nassau airport to Sandals Royal Bahamian Resort and Spa — a AAA Five Diamond award winner, no less — and by 10 a.m. you're reclining poolside with a rum punch in hand. And there's the added bonus of gallivanting about all day with no money or credit cards weighing down your string bikini.

LOCATION

Nassau, the Bahamian capital, is a city rich in blue skies, turquoise waters, history and personality. Since its founding in 1656, on through its flirtations with colonialism, piracy, rum smuggling and currently tourism, it has always been the nucleus of the 700 islands that make up the Bahamas. The resort is on the white-sand Cable Beach.

DESIGN

The rooms are certainly conducive to the ways of *l'amour* — their design hearkens back to the resort's colonial beginnings (it later became a favourite vacation spot for the Windsors). Despite the days-gone-by décor of the suites, there are enough modern-day amenities to make any third-millennium vacationer positively blissful.

But instead of the satellite TV, high-tech air conditioning and so forth, let's talk about the king-size mahogany four-poster bed. It's high and expansive and movie-set gorgeous. Crisp white linens, double-sized pillows — it's this sort of attention to detail that sets the deluxe apart from the mediocre.

And the Ultra Spa follows suit. It routinely makes the top ten list of spa resorts in *Condé Nast Traveler's* reader survey, in part for its Roman-influenced décor. There are Corinthian columns in the lobby, as well as a carved stone fountain, and walls and floors of Italian Satumia stone. The curved reception counter and doors are dark mahogany; pre-Raphaelite artwork comes in gilded frames; and the hot-and-cold plunge pools out front are undeniably toga-worthy.

CLIENTELE

The Sandals slogan is "Love is all you need," and that's precisely what you will need to gain admittance into this ultra-inclusive couples-only resort (as '70s as that sounds). But there are loads of couples who take vacations together, so the mood is more raucous than you'd expect. Men frequent the Ultra Spa almost as much as the women, many taking advantage of the ever-popular Couples Massages and Massage Duet, wherein you learn the art of the massage from professionals, then practise on your partner in the comfort of your ocean-front suite.

TREATMENTS

The smell of eucalyptus greets you as you enter the well-appointed spa. From facials that use therapeutic plant extracts and traditional natural remedies (like the seaweed or Sun Lover's facials), to body mud masques (excellent for holiday side effects like skin inflammation or sunburn), to the Desert Heat Body Wrap (contains elements like copper, magnesium and zinc to help hydrate and tone your vacationing bod), this Sandals brand Ultra Spa is clearly no resort afterthought. They use the Pevonia spa product and sun protection line, made from pure botanical extracts.

And what better way to relieve the body of several layers of dead winter cells than a Salt Glo? You're given a robe and a smile, and before long you're lying buck naked on a towel-draped massage table, head down in a face cradle. The thirty-five-minute scrub is immensely enjoyable and useful, and you'll emerge soft as a kitten — purring, too. Afterwards, you can stop into the salon for a few braids for that full-on "I was in the Bahamas and you weren't" mien.

NEARBY

With all of the water and land sports, gourmet restaurants, fitness classes and frozen poolside Mudslides to be had at the resort, you won't likely feel the need to leave. But if you do, start with their private offshore island, Sandals Cay, for a little getaway from your getaway (included in the all-inclusive deal). It boasts its own swim-up pool bar, Caribbean restaurant and buttery beaches.

Venturing into greater Nassau, the Doongalik Studios are an art gallery cum sculpture garden cum souvenir shop that has also taken on the task of organizing Junkanoo. That's the colourful annual celebration that began during the sixteenth and seventeenth centuries, when slaves were allowed to leave the plantations at Christmastime to celebrate the holidays with African dance, music and costumes. This tradition continues today in a firecracker of a parade held on Boxing Day and again on New Year's Day.

The so-called Fish Fry district along Cable Beach is where you'll find authentic conch shacks, like Goldie's, that offer up the crustaceans in every form imaginable, including deep-fried crack conch, conch fritters and ceviche-style marinated conch salad.

The covered Straw Market (located just down the street from the British Colonial Hilton Hotel) is teeming with colourful hand-woven baskets, dolls, drums, shakers and assorted knick-knacks.

184

SERVICE

Friendly beyond compare.

BOTTOM LINE

When you inevitably find yourself winging your way back to Canada, all bronzed and buffed, you may find that you're not yet ready to leave your all-inclusive vacation behind. So grab some duty-free rum at the airport and mix up a batch of Bahama Mamas once you settle back into your abode. Then, take heart as you listen to the wind howling outside. After all, there's always next weekend.

INFORMATION

Sandals Royal Bahamian Resort & Spa. Cable Beach, Nassau, Bahamas.
Phone: 1-800-545-8282 or (242) 327-6400. Web: http://www.sandals.com.
The Salt Glo (US$50) and other spa treatments are not included in the signing price.

Photo by Amy Rosen

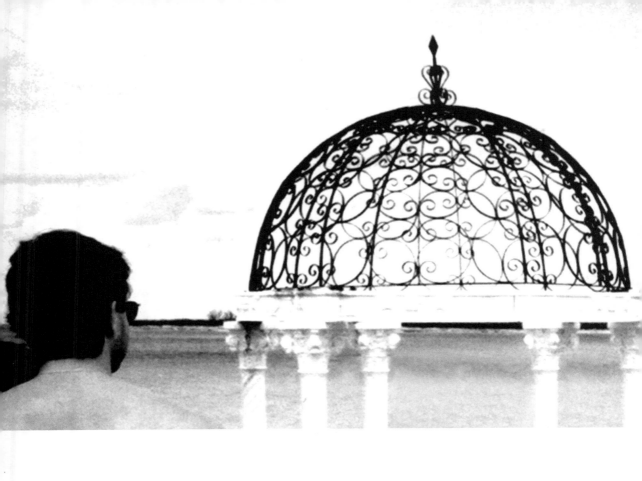

SPATOPIA

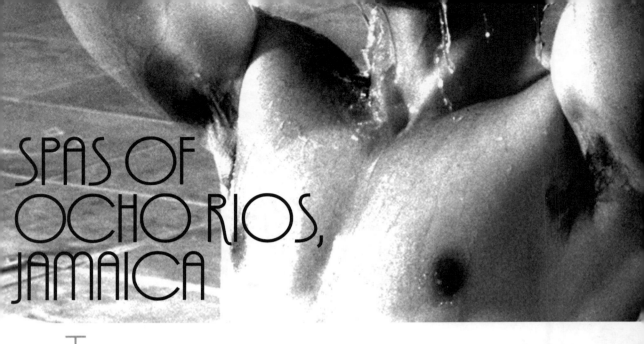

SPAS OF OCHO RIOS, JAMAICA

There's nothing like escaping a Canadian winter for warmer climes — that welcome blast of steamy air upon deplaning, your first glimpse of a palm tree, folks clad in bikinis instead of balaclavas. The islands beckon, and the tropical town of Ocho Rios trumpets more loudly than most. Known as the garden of Jamaica, it's a place where the locals say heaven spills into the sea.

Set amidst a lush landscape of rolling green mountains, sandy coves and craggy coastlines, Ocho Rios is also the birthplace of Jamaica's favourite son, Bob Marley. And next to Marley's music, the best way to feel all right is to take advantage of the biggest thing to happen here since reggae: Jamaica's burgeoning spa industry. All the new hotels have them, the older ones are building them, and the best fuse the natural environs with a healthy dose of island spirituality.

LOCATION

Tucked into the north coast of Jamaica, Ocho Rios is a two-hour drive from the Montego Bay airport. Upon landing at nearby Discovery Bay in 1494, Christopher Columbus described the area as "the fairest land mine eyes have ever seen," and visitors might think likewise during the winding drive in. The majority of the spas are about a ten-minute drive from the city centre.

TREATMENTS

There are three ways to do spas in Ocho Rios: all-inclusive properties where treatments are included; all-inclusive properties where spa treatments cost extra; and boutique hotels with spas. Each offers distinctly different experiences.

The Sans Souci Resort and Spa, a AAA Four Diamond Award winner, is an ultra-inclusive resort where gourmet food, fruity drinks, activities, spa treatments and even weddings are included in the package price. Charlie's Spa (so named for the enormous sea turtle that lives in a grotto on site) is set into a wooded bluff overlooking the Caribbean, and is also home to a natural mineral spring, one of four in the region. The outdoor Jacuzzi has a tropical canopy of ferns, hanging vines and coconut trees, and the natural mineral pool is full of potassium, sodium, calcium and magnesium, great for soothing skin and calming nerves. Most of the treatment rooms are open-air cabanas with names like "Hideaway" (a fave for couples massages).

The spa offers a good range of facials, wraps, reflexology and the like. Five treatments are included with a full-price booking, but unfortunately they're only thirty minutes long and quite superficial. On the other hand, they provide an easy way for timid newbies to get a taste of spa living, and all services can be expanded to a full hour for an extra charge. The no-tipping policy is a bonus.

The Royal Plantation Spa and Golf Resort is also an award-winning, ultra-inclusive property, with a new spa decked out in elegant, plantation-style décor. The waiting area is scented by eucalyptus wafting in from the steam room and is stocked with sweet Jamaican spring water and comfy chairs while you fill out the health questionnaire. "Have you had food in the past two hours?" Yes — conch fritters, jerk chicken, mango, pumpkin rice, ackee and saltfish, rum fruitcake and a pineapple. "Have you had alcohol in the past four hours?" Um, yes: two strawberry daiquiris, a piña colada, a Hummingbird and a Red Stripe beer. (What do they expect? This is all-inclusive!)

Aside from being offered drinks from the bar while luxuriating in the hydrotherapy tub, there is little difference between this spa and a high-end North American one — which is nice, but also a little disappointing. One would hope for more authentic Jamaican treatments using local traditions. However, the Beaches' signature spa products — lemongrass-infused creams, teas, candles and oils — are all locally produced. Added bonus: the staff call you "M'Lady."

The KiYara Ocean Spa is located on the grounds of the Jamaica Inn, an exquisite forty-five-room hotel that Winston Churchill, Noel Coward and Ian Fleming frequented back in the day. Newly opened in August 2002, the KiYara is the epitome of a spa paradise. Its name means "sacred place of the earth spirits" in the language of the Taino Indians, the original inhabitants of this area.

All treatments are based on indigenous ingredients, many of which are grown just outside the spa and are used seasonally, akin to the ways owner Carolyn Jobson's ancestors used them to nurture spirit and soul. The KiYara spa is carved into a hillside that overlooks the Caribbean, its relaxation deck and massage tables open to warm sun rays and soft sea breezes. By night, there's moonlight yoga and meditation.

The look of the place is *Flintstones* chic: a seven-headed Vichy shower fashioned out of bamboo, rustic thatched roofs, walls of woven branches, local art and fabrics.

Treatments range from a barefoot Fijian massage and Taino Opia stone massage (which uses warm river stones from the island) to the Blue Mountain coffee toner. This hour-long treatment is meant to pull and flush toxins from the body, speed up cellular metabolism and help break down cellulite. It starts with Jobson saying a little prayer, then leads into a coffee-and-clay-mask exfoliation, a quick bake under the sun, and a rinse under an outdoor shower. Back on the massage table, there's a rehydrating rub of honey, lime and essential oils, and finally an incredible lymph-drainage massage. Lime-tinged water is imbibed throughout, with a spicy ginger and cucumber beverage offered at the end.

BOTTOM LINE

Spas that embrace local ingredients and traditions, and celebrate Jamaica's gorgeous land-scape, are spas you've got to love. A tropical rubdown in an island paradise? Irie, mon!

INFORMATION

Sans Souci Resort and Spa. Phone: 1-800-448-7702 or (876) 994-1206. Web: http://www.sanssoucijamaica.com.

Royal Plantation Spa and Golf Resort. Phone: 1-888-48-ROYAL (1-888-487-6925). Web: http://www.royalplantation.com.

KiYara Ocean Spa at Jamaica Inn. Phone: (876) 974-2380 (Jamaica Inn phone: 1-800-837-4600, and Web: http://www.jamaicainn.com).

Ocho Rios Tourist Board. Phone: (876) 974-2582.

SPA AT THE FOUR SEASONS RESORT, URUGUAY

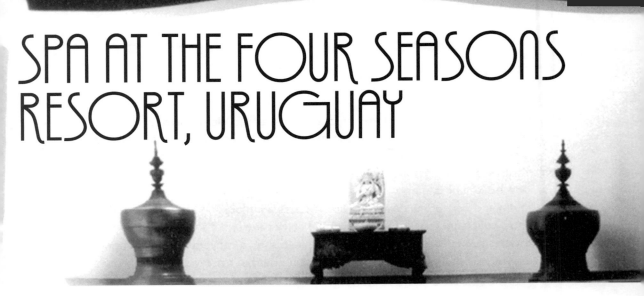

The east-meets-west philosophy found at many of today's spas couples the swank modern ideals of North American city-dwellers with the calming presence of nature-infused environs. But what happens when east meets south, as it does at the spa at the Four Seasons Resort in Carmelo? For one thing, innovative treatments that use indigenous ingredients like Uruguayan wines and eucalyptus honey to delicious effect. For another, sumptuous surroundings carved out of the wilderness on the banks of the Rio de la Plata. But what's best is that this spa incorporates all of those famous Four Seasons touches along with more reasonable South American pricing, guaranteeing you the vacation of a lifetime with pocket change to spare.

LOCATION

After a brief twenty-minute flight (or two-hour scenic boat trip on the Rio de la Plata) from Buenos Aires, ceramic tumblers filled with lemongrass iced tea welcome you to the resort in Uruguay. Nestled against the winding river, among sturdy pine and eucalyptus forests, free-range cattle ranches and rolling green plains, the setting is elegant and serene. Boardwalks guide you around the half-rugged, half-manicured landscape. The area is also a South American playground offering horseback riding, water sports, a visit to the nearby town of Colonia (a UNESCO World Heritage Site) or an evening at the neighbouring 100-year-old Narbona House, where sublime red wines are made from the vineyards surrounding the resort.

DESIGN

The Four Seasons' forty-four expansive bi-level suites and private bungalows have cathedral ceilings and are crafted from South American Lapacho and Viraro wood. The Asian-influenced décor incorporates heated slate floors, outdoor garden showers and wood-burning fireplaces with all the modern amenities one could imagine. Even when the hotel is fully booked, the layout is such that you feel completely secluded. The three-tiered waterfall pool is a focal point of the property; it's vast and gorgeous (and staff come by with free gelato when it's hot outside!). The par-72 golf course, meanwhile, has been called the best on the continent. The spa is in step with the resort's overall Asian vibe — it's all fountains and meditation in a yin-and-yang-meets-gaucho kind of way. There is a handful of treatment rooms (named Earth, Air, Water, Spirit and Fire), a fully equipped exercise room and an aerobics, yoga and meditation studio where free classes are held daily (in English and Spanish).

Photo by Amy Rosen

CLIENTELE

Singles, couples, friends, families. A lot of moneyed Brits and Americans who work in Buenos Aires and hit upon the resort because of the Four Seasons name.

TREATMENTS

An innovative lineup of hydrotherapy, massages, facials and nail care. Whatever you come for, it starts with choosing a fortune at the front desk (one must assume they're all good). Then it's off to the lovely change room, before getting down to business in one of the candlelit treatment rooms. If you decide upon an Asian Blend massage, the therapist will have you select a Tarot-style card that might say something like "Efficiency." Interesting. Then she'll point to a bowl of smooth, coloured stones and ask you to choose one. Very interesting. Then she'll go to work on you — quite *efficiently*, mind you — working out any stress and knots that somehow weren't released during your morning walk, yoga class, midday swim *or* afternoon snooze. At the end of it all, you'll drink a glass of water that contains your chosen crystal (in my case, amethyst), being careful not to swallow the semi-precious gem. Since little English is spoken in the spa (many of the therapists are well-trained locals), most of the New Age touches go unexplained. But no matter; it still amounts to as Zen-like an experience as you'll have without converting.

SERVICE

Discreet without being snooty. It's the perfect gelling of the outgoing South American personality with patented Four Seasons hospitality. You want a hearty handshake and a welcoming back slap? They'll do that for you. You want all eyes averted and to be left alone? They can do that, too. Yoga instructor Dianne is a sweet and powerful pixie from Ontario who is married to the resort's head chef, Thomas Bellec, formerly of Truffles in Toronto. Thomas gave a great little cooking class, and also cooked up a favourite dinner in the smart Pura restaurant, which featured free-range Argentine beef cooked on the classic asado grill. Charbroiled never tasted *this* good, especially when coupled with the finest local Malbec wines.

BOTTOM LINE

When it's winter in Canada, it's summer in Uruguay. Remember that as you recline on the terry-cloth-covered loungers by the waterfall pool, snacking on homemade *dulce de leche* cookies after a day of horseback riding, a South American beat massage at the spa and a mediation session. Little wonder the Four Seasons Carmelo was selected one of the fifty-two best new hotels in the world in 2002 by *Condé Nast Traveler*, as well as earning every other accolade in the business. They really are that good.

INFORMATION

Four Seasons Resort, Carmelo, Uruguay. Phone: 011-598-542-9000. Web: http://www.fourseasons.com/carmelo. Deals at the resort include round-trip private plane ride, three nights in a deluxe bungalow, gourmet buffet break-fast, unlimited golf and access to all amenities for around US$1,000 a person. The Asian Blend massage lasted 55 minutes and cost $80.

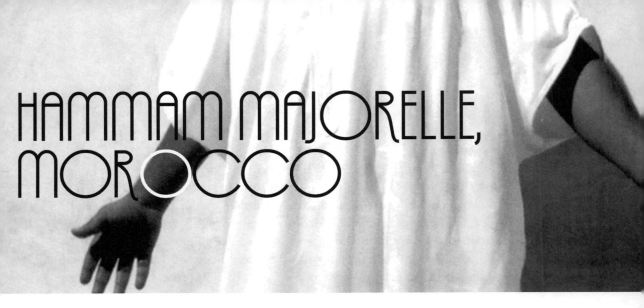

HAMMAM MAJORELLE, MOROCCO

Stretched out in a sun-parched valley swathed in groves of date trees and palms lies Marrakesh, a storybook come to life. It's a city where snake charmers and acrobats enchant the throngs within Jemaa el-Fna Square, the epicentre of the exotic walled city. Donkeys pulling rickety carts kick up dirt while manoeuvring through a web of centuries-old paths and archways, passing market stalls fuelled by carpet hawkers, honeyed pastries and preserved lemons.

One could be happy here in southern Morocco to do little more than hoof around the cobblestones, eat lamb brains and have a monkey tossed onto your shoulders for a $10 photo op every now and again. But you haven't been to Marrakesh until you have experienced the Arabic spa treatment known as the *hammam*. These are public bath houses, a progression of hot, quiet, watery rooms where naked strangers scrub you within an inch of your life as part of a weekly ritual that keeps Moroccans looking clean and sprightly. And it's the perfect vehicle to get that travellers' dust and stink out of your pores.

LOCATION

As the Islamic faith spread, so did the hammam; many are still standing in Iran, Asia and across North Africa from Egypt to Morocco. Like the Roman baths of yesteryear, the hammam was a place to socialize, and entrance fees were a mere pittance so that everyone could enjoy. Hammam Majorelle is in the same Marrakesh neighbourhood as Jardin Majorelle, fashion designer Yves Saint-Laurent's famously lush garden, but you can find good hammams in resort spas, grimy markets, and every nook and cranny of high- and low-end quarters. Guidebooks and tourist offices can suggest some good ones, or ask a friendly local to take you to his or her favourite.

DESIGN

Subterranean torture-chamber chic. Sleepy dim lighting, white subway tile with black accents. Arched doorways, three rooms of varying steamy temperatures, plastic water buckets, silver taps, a disposable razor floating by. Water, water, everywhere.

CLIENTELE

The hammam is a public forum where very intimate things happen. A woman bathes her child, a group of teenagers meticulously scrub each other, a trio of petrified Brits in bikinis mull over whether to take the plunge. It's a cross-section of society taking an hour out of a hectic day to take care of their bodies. When Mohammed first advocated the use of the hammam (the word is Arabic for "spreader of warmth"), women were forbidden because he believed the procedure enhanced fertility. But as the hygienic benefits became apparent, the rule was relaxed and women were

Photo by Amy Rosen

permitted, albeit only after an illness or giving birth. It wasn't long, however, before the hammam privilege became a right, to the point that if a husband denied his wife her weekly visits, she had grounds for divorce.

TREATMENTS

There are two choices at the hammam: do it yourself or have someone do it to you. For the latter, you arrive with a towel and a loofah mitt you bought in the market for under a buck. Pay $7 at the entrance and make your way into the forbidding tomb. Strip down to nothing. Wrap your arms around yourself for comfort and modesty as you take a seat — on the slippery tile floor or a tiny plastic bench that goes from one bare bottom to the next without any cleansing (not the most hygienic place, but when in Rome…).

At this point, an oversized Moroccan woman (or man, if you're on the men's side, which is separate but identical in form and function), takes you by the wrist and forces you to the ground on your back (she knows no English, so each step goes from one shock to the next). Donning your loofah mitt, she attacks you with olive oil soap and unforgiving hands. This special soap contains extracts from black olives and is combined with the native Argan oil, which is full of vitamin E. Her zeal is unrelenting. The subsequent scrubbing of the body can best be described as a pleasant pain; it makes you wince, but you know it's doing you good, and the chunks of eraser-like bits that were formerly your skin further attest to that.

The scrubbing stops. You take a moment to recover while she works over your neighbour, but before long she's scooping a handful of thick olive oil cream from a tub and slapping it on the wet tiled wall. Suddenly, she's upon you again, twisting your right arm and forcing you back to the floor, this time facedown. You like her better this time because she's massaging you with dollops of rich cream from the wall and is actually smiling a bit. You slide around the wet floor, like a greased pig; she continues to rub you hard, crack your joints, then dumps a bucket of cold water over your head with aplomb. You're done.

BOTTOM LINE

From wealthy tourists to the working class, hammams are the great equalizer of the spa world. They may not be fancy, but they're good clean fun.

INFORMATION

If you bring your own bucket, special soap, stool and mitt, the hammam costs about 60 cents. Otherwise, prices range from $5 to $18 at high-end spas. Hammam Majorelle is located at Cartier Gueliz, Marrakesh, near Jardin Majorelle. Or try Hammam Dar el-Bacha, 20 Rue Fatima Zohra, Medina, behind Jemaa el-Fna Square; or Hammam Safi, Boulevarde de Safi, Gueliz, near Jardin Majorelle.

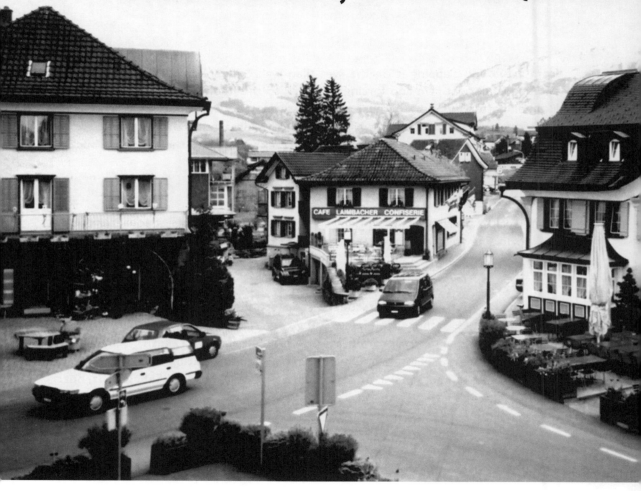

HOF WEISSBAD, SWITZERLAND

Thought to be the domain of the wealthy and fabulous, jetting to a spa in Switzerland conjures up images of trophy wives and Elton John being buffed with essential oils and swathed in Egyptian linens.

But don't be fooled: Swiss spas offer tough love. Most have more in common with the clinical vibe of a rehab facility than the cozy North American spas upon which many of us were weaned. That's why the Swiss call them "wellness hotels" and "health spas." Think healing, not indulgence; hospital sheets, not white Frette towels; silence, not New Age soundtrack.

Even so, Hof Weissbad, in the heart of the tiny town of Weissbad in the Appenzell region of eastern Switzerland, has an appealing roster of excellent treatments — not to mention the regal looks and demeanour of a decadent wellness retreat from the 1920s. The exterior of the eighty-five-room four-star spa and rehabilitation centre is all pale yellows, striped awnings and white wicker. In front, a sprawling veranda overlooks a wildflower garden and the mountains of the Alpstein, making it the perfect spot for a sun-dappled lunch of Appenzell cheese and spring asparagus salad.

Inside, however, the spa is crisp and sterile and it means business.

Photo by Amy Rosen

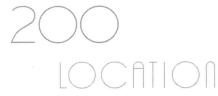

LOCATION

An hour from cosmopolitan Zurich via Swiss-timed trains, the backdrop is the Alpstein, where three mountain chains rise up from lovely market towns. Appenzell, a small hamlet of brightly painted gingerbread houses and cobblestone walkways, is just minutes away. Appenzellers pride themselves on their heritage of crafts (they call them "living traditions"), and shop windows are adorned with colourful works of needlepoint and intricate pieces of woodworking and silver. Refreshingly, this handiwork isn't meant for strolling tourists, but rather for proud locals to decorate their homes. There's also an extensive network of hiking paths, Alpine skiing and natural springs in nearby Heiden, where people come from afar for the healing attributes of its warm water.

DESIGN

Living quarters are comfortable but utilitarian, featuring Ikea-style soft, down duvet–covered beds with televisions and spacious baths. White tiles (with a line of pretty wave accents), cold massage tables and water hoses abound in the spa treatment rooms. The Zen-inspired quiet room adjacent to the outdoor and indoor pools, and the exercise room, with its wooden floor and wall of windows, are warm and inviting. Such new additions as the subterranean steam, shower and sauna rooms are contemporary and calming with mosaic blues and cedar accents.

CLIENTELE

Hof Weissbad is the well-bred choice of upper-crust and aging Swiss who come to stay to recuperate from an operation or illness. The spa's clinical department is a private hospital recognized by the cantonal department of health and is considered a rehabilitation clinic. With private nurses and five-star dining on site, it has snob appeal up the Appenzell. But it's also a popular retreat for Euro-chic mother-and-daughter teams and a popular getaway for team-building conferences. North Americans are few and far between.

TREATMENTS

Many visitors are here to get better. Here's the drill: Get naked! Bend over! Crawl into the *Dauerbrause*! There's no translation for the German word *Dauerbrause*, but imagine a huge iron lung that leaves only your head exposed and contains a moving rainstorm that massages and cleanses every crevice of your body with alternating warm and cold gushes of water. Looks scary but feels womb-like.

With a little yellow schedule card dotted with words like *Meersalzbad*, *Wassergymnastik* and *Korperpeeling*, one never knows exactly what to expect, which makes it hilarious when you're anticipating a soothing massage but are instead met by an oversized aesthetician brandishing a paintbrush loaded with ice-cold algae. The house specialty is thalassotherapy — treatments that use a combination of algae, massage, turbo tubs and local mineral waters that leave you bright-eyed and invigorated.

FOOD & DRINK

Breakfasts are a smorgasbord of freshly baked breads, local cheeses, cured meats, meusli, yogurt and fresh and stewed fruits that will often carry you through to dinner. Dinner may be an intriguing caraway soup, pan-fried trout sided by crisp rosti, or beef filet and roast potatoes, with gingerbread parfait for dessert (the region is big on all things gingerbread). A good wine list features French and Italian picks. Top off the meal with another local specialty, Alpenbitter on ice. Made from forty-two different herbs, it has a floral edge reminiscent of Jägermeister, but the medicinal kick of Buckley's Mixture.

SERVICE

The staff is pleasant, professional and efficient, but if you don't speak German, the language barrier can at times be an issue. Be prepared to talk loudly and use sweeping hand motions, or learn German fast.

BOTTOM LINE

At times it's too cold or too hot, but in the end you leave beautiful Switzerland relaxed and rejuvenated, albeit with a belly full of cheese, wine and chocolate.

INFORMATION

Hotel Hof Weissbad. 9057 Weissbad, Weissbad, Switzerland. Phone: 011-41-71-798-80-80. Web: http://www.hofweissbad.ch, or e-mail hotel@hofweissbad.ch. Standard rooms start at US$230 per night.

SPA HOPPING IN SWITZERLAND

The abundance of natural hot springs in the eastern part of Switzerland has given rise to a host of rehabilitation centres and wellness hotels. In the towns of Heiden and Bad Ragaz, for example, you can take in the springs, visit an old-school spa and even stop in at one of the new deluxe operations, all for about what you'd pay for comparable treatments in North America.

Plus, they've got all of that great scenery going for them. And, of course, there's the chocolate.

HEIDEN

Heiden is about a two-hour train ride from Zurich, an enjoyable trip that offers panoramic views. Hotel Heiden, a top Swiss wellness hotel and spa, is set above sparkly Lake Constance. You can take in some fresh air by hiking around the well-marked nature paths that wind around the town and into the mountains. Or climb the steps of the bell tower for a sweeping look over Heiden and the lake, with Germany and Austria off in the distance. The best treatments at Hotel Heiden include a Fichtennadelbad massage, which is basically a tried-and-true therapeutic Swedish massage. The Chi Yang Schonheits massage, however, is a knockout facial that uses a combination of essential oils, masks, scented steam and experienced hands. It is more than ninety minutes in duration and is so consuming that it makes your head feel like an entity all its own, floating magically above the rest of your body.

Also located in Heiden is Heilbad Unterrechstein, a woodsy bathhouse and fitness centre where the water is spring-fed and warm. People come from afar for its healing powers. You can drink the water cold, and many people do, but consider yourself forewarned: the high sulphur content makes it taste like rotten eggs.

BAD RAGAZ

About a forty-minute drive from Heiden is Bad Ragaz. Recently branded Heidiland by the local tourist commission, Bad Ragaz is famous for the children's story about a vivacious little girl, Heidi, and her friend the goat boy. Situated 510 metres above sea level in the Rhine valley, the resort town — "where wild waters work wonders" — has a hot spring that gushes from Tamina Gorge. The gorge was discovered in 1038, but it was not until two hundred years later that local monks made good use of the warm water's purported healing powers.

Today, the town thrives on spa culture, and at its core is a public bath-house called Tamina Therme. This slick, modern building is home to one open-air and two indoor pools — in which the water is 34 degrees Celsius — with a waterfall, bubble-massage seats and massage jets. When you emerge from the buoyant waters, a woman dressed in hospital whites wraps you in a warm sheet. Such is the healing spa aesthetic in Switzerland.

With its ritzy hotels and high-priced shops, Bad Ragaz attracts a wealthy clientele. No doubt many of them visit the beautiful new Ad Fontes spa, home to the plush terry-cloth robes and towels for which you may be yearning. The featured treatment here is the Hay Bed, in which you're painted with cold algae, rolled up straitjacket-style in a sheet and laid in an honest-to-goodness bed of hay to let the body mask work its wonders. An hour later, you awake detoxified — and feeling comatose.

ELSEWHERE

For the best in Swiss outdoor activities, there's biking, hiking and boating in the summer, endless downhill and cross-country ski routes in the winter, great home-grown cuisine, including crisp potato rosti and pan-fried trout, and fine local wines from this burgeoning vine region.

Gesundes Wissen, a drug store with a difference in Heiden, has a naturo-pathic doctor on staff and a herb garden out back. They prepare personalized potions, lotions, pills and powders in their basement laboratory.

The closest you'll come to a city outside of Zurich is St. Gallen, a half-hour bus ride from Heiden. It has all the name-brand stores you would expect — including, yes, a McDonald's. Make a beeline for the famous Bucherer jewellery shop, where you will have little trouble supporting the Swiss economy.

BOTTOM LINE

These postcard-perfect towns of eastern Switzerland were built around hot springs and therapeutic spa culture, so they know what they're doing. So what if most of the springs are a tad sterile — they're also healing. And what does it matter if the spa aestheticians hose you down while yelling at you in German? It only makes the experience that much more memorable.

INFORMATION

Hotel Heiden. Phone: 011-41-71-898-1515. Web: http://www.hotelheiden.ch.
Heilbad Unterrechstein. Phone: 011-41-71-898-3388. Web: http://www.heilbad.ch.
Tamina Therme. Phone: 011-41-81-303-3030.
Ad Fontes. Phone: 011-41-81-302-4010.

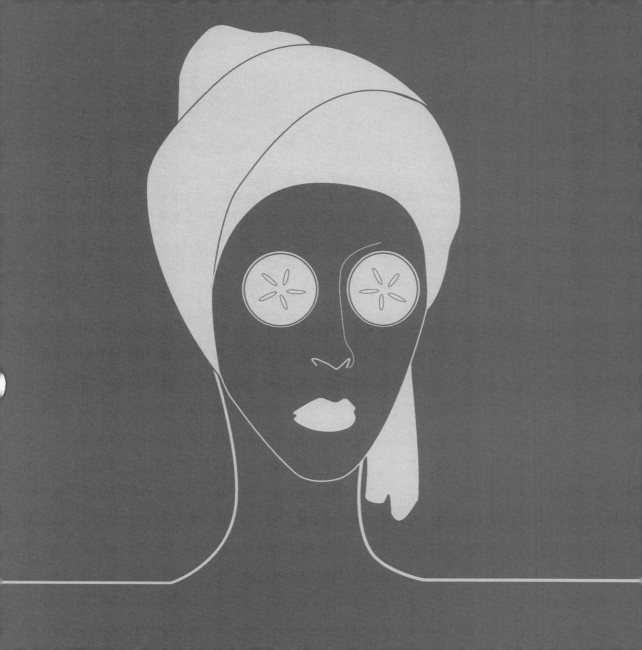

AIRPORT SPAS

AIRPORT SPAS

Toronto's new Terminal 1 has opened to well-deserved fanfare for its gorgeous artwork, such as suspended silhouettes and a tank filled with floating cubes. But what, no spa?

That's a bit of a missed opportunity, since flight delays and cancellations have aided a proliferation of airport spas around the globe. In fact, a recent poll in *Business Traveler* magazine revealed that almost 60 percent of respondents would visit an airport spa if given the chance. So say goodbye to catnaps on coffee-stained terminal floors, and treat yourself instead to an anti-swelling leg massage, a hit of pre-boarding oxygen therapy, or one of the other treatments available at the following airport spas.

Vancouver

Absolute Spa at the Fairmont Vancouver Airport hotel was the first in line for take off in North America, offering a full slate of by-appointment services including Ayurvedic oil treatments, hot-stone massages and gentlemen's facials. The idea is that if you're stuck in the airport for a layover anyway, you might as well make the most of it in sumptuous West Coast surroundings.

But if you find yourself at YVR with just an extra hour to spare, don't fret — just head over to one of the other two Absolute branches in the terminal. At the domestic gates, the little open nook of a spa specializes in treatments that help counter the negative effects of air travel. (The second location is near the U.S. departure gates.)

Joey, a registered massage therapist, gave me an anti-swelling leg massage for twenty minutes, then I had a thirty-minute Tailwinds Express manicure, and finally rubber tubing was stuck up my nose for a ten-minute burst of citrus-scented oxygen. Within the span of an hour, I had all but prevented potentially life-threatening deep-vein thrombosis, had a pair of moist mitts, and the oxygen helped to boost my immune system for that stale cabin air.

Open daily from 9 a.m. to 7 p.m.
For more information, visit http://www.absolutespa.com.

Bangkok

The first massage I ever had took place on the beach in Thailand. I was attacked from behind, slathered in coconut oil and twisted into a sandy pretzel. I couldn't walk for the next two days, but that's what you get in a place where massage is a way of life — everyone thinks he's an expert. And at Lek Foot Massage at Bangkok's Don Muang airport, they are. Rows of black leather chairs and a squadron of masseuses offer brawny Thai massages or, for the more timid, reflexology. Almost as good as joining the mile-high club.

Next to Gate 15, on the departures level.
For more information, visit http://www.airportthai.co.th.

Calgary

Again, Canadians were ahead of the curve as Calgary's OraOxygen Spa was the world's first airport-based oxygen wellness spa. Founder Suzanne Letourneau, a former flight attendant, came up with the concept during a particularly exhausting four-hour layover. Although she started out in early 2000 focusing on the benefits of fresh oxygen (relieves headaches, boosts energy, calms the nervous system and improves sleep), the spa also offers the full roster of massages, wraps, facials, nail treatments and even ear candling to help ease the pain that can come with flying at high altitudes. Satellite spa locations have since opened in the new McNamara Terminal of Detroit's Metro Airport and Amsterdam's Schiphol Airport (where you'll also find the Back to Life massage chairs in the departures area between gates E and F).

Located on the second floor behind the Air Canada check-in desks. Open from 7 a.m. to 9 p.m.
For more information, visit http://www.oraoxygen.net.

London

The luxe Molton Brown Travel Spa provides complimentary spa treatments exclusively to British Airways customers travelling in its First and Club World classes, as well as BA Executive Club gold cardholders. Therapies last from ten to fifteen minutes and range from reflex therapies for the hands and feet that use crystal dynamics and the acupressure reflex technique, to circulation therapies meant to realign the flow of energies via oriental head and shoulder massages. If no staff members are immediately available, a pager is given to clients and they're buzzed when a therapist becomes free. On your own time, special steam suites and body jet hydrotherapy showers soothe, clean and tone via aquamassage.

Located in the Terminal 1 and Terminal 4 departures lounges at Heathrow.
For more information, visit http://www.moltonbrown.co.uk.

Miami

There's no spa per se, but a dip in the palm-flanked pool and a run on the jogging track at the Miami International Airport Hotel's eighth-floor health club will make you feel like a million bucks. There's also a whirlpool beside the alfresco rooftop pool, where snacks and cocktails are served. The steely locker room is useful after a sauna, workout or racquetball game, and the club can provide necessities such as racquets and safety goggles. The club hosts a mélange of air travellers and airport personnel. It's a three-star hotel, so don't expect it to win any beauty contests, but it's right in the terminal, providing easy access to good clean fun.

Open daily from 6 a.m. to 10 p.m.
For more information, visit http://www.miahotel.com.

Newark

The D_parture Spa is a sleek outfit that's all blond wood and cheeky graphics. On offer are manicures, quick fixes of oxygen therapy and even high-flying packages such as the Weary Traveler, which includes a pedicure with heated massage, paraffin and a little lie-down to ease jet lag. Facials include makeup removal and "targeted moisturizing" designed for air travel. The first D_parture Spa was such a hit that a second branch has been added in Terminal B near the duty-free shop.

Open daily in Terminal C, beside Gate 92, from 7 a.m. to 8:30 p.m., and in Terminal B from 10 a.m. to 8 p.m.
For more information, visit http://www.departurespa.com.

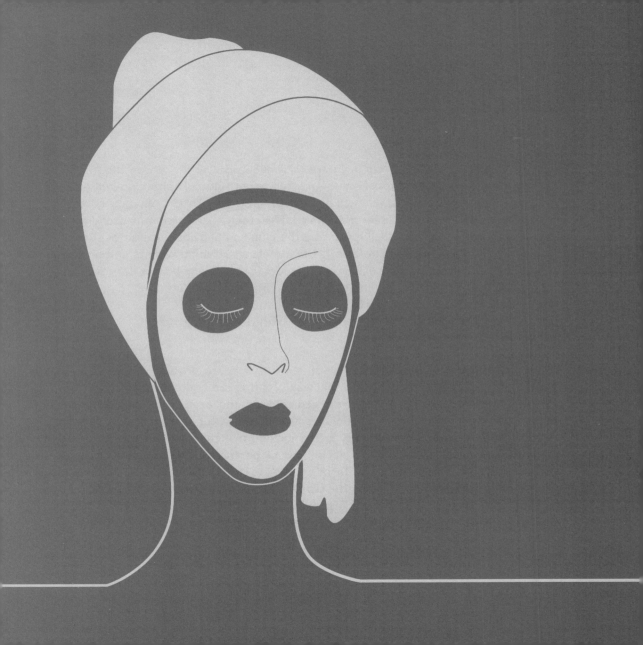

SPAS FOR SENIORS

SPAS FOR SENIORS

My grandmother, Fran Salem, and her younger sister Marion Rossman are going to the spa. To be precise, they're hitting **HealthWinds Spa**, a chic health and wellness spa in uptown Toronto, for a Reflexology Foot Massage and a Hydradermie Facial.

Considering that both women are octogenarians — one with a heart condition, the other with osteoporosis — they're not exactly the variety of spa-goer you would imagine prancing around earth-tone rooms wearing terry-cloth robes. But think again, because after women and men in their twenties and thirties, senior citizens constitute the next fastest growing demographic in the spa market, says Kailee Kline, president of a thirty-one-member association called Spas Ontario and the owner of HealthWinds.

And, she explains, this makes sense. "Although our primary market is younger, we have been getting more calls from senior citizens, and they're not at all shy about telling us that they're senior citizens, and are also quick to point out that they have all sorts of health ailments."

Situated in a medical building at Yonge Street and Eglinton Avenue, HealthWinds takes a lot of referrals from physicians in the area. The Ontario government health plan doesn't cover these services, but many, including massage, are covered by extended health benefit plans.

Kline believes that there has been a shift in attitude among the aged. "Ten years ago, senior citizens would have considered these treatments frivolous, but now people are realizing, 'You know what? I'm here for the long term and I want to feel good while I'm here.'"

Back at HealthWinds, reflexologist Giovanna and aesthetician Elena lead Fran and Marion into the change room. At first, the grandmothers insist on wearing the robes over their street clothes (too much of a hassle to undress), but in time they concede. Swimming in terry cloth and sipping lemon-tinged water, they sit in the airy relaxation room, with its blond hardwood floors, fireplace and comfy chairs, questioning the expediency of listing all of their medications on the official health form.

Fran ends up jotting down "loads" while Marion writes "too many." (Their various afflictions had been discussed with Kline ahead of time). "You know, when you're young, you take it all for granted because your body is beautiful to start with," Fran pontificates. "But when you get older, you really need to take care of things. It's like maintenance with a car."

And with that, she's off to her treatment room.

Anne Anderson of the **Spa at Hockley Valley Resort** near Orangeville, Ontario, says her spa has also seen a steady increase in senior spa clients over the past few years, and estimates that they now represent about 20 percent of her business. "They like the manicures and pedicures, but we actually have a group of five in right now and they're getting the works: massages, facials, scrubs, manicures and pedicures."

Anderson says that some of the treatments do elevate body temperatures, so clients should inform the spa of any health concerns before booking treatments.

The aged spa-goer isn't just looking for pretty nails and stress reduction; they also are interested in health maintenance. HealthWinds' Kline says spas must determine what kinds of treatments are safe, and also effective. If clients are taking heart medications such as Coumadin (an anticoagulant), for example, it would prohibit a spa from performing massage therapy, hydrotherapy or anything else that would accelerate the circulation. Of course, yet another important aspect of visiting a spa, for young and old alike, is having treatments that are enjoyable. So, for Marion, Kline chose a facial, a service that is both soothing and designed to treat aging skin. Fran also wanted something hands-on, but because of her history of heart disease, a regular massage wasn't an option.

Reflexology, however, was. "It focuses on working the pressure points of the feet, the head and the hands," Kline says. "The theory behind it is that by pressing these different points you free blockages that are interconnected to various parts. So, in a sense, we are actually working the whole body through these points, and it's soothing as well." Pressure can be varied to suit age and tastes, from light or medium to strong or even vigorous.

After about an hour, my aunt and grandmother emerge from their treatments looking more relaxed than I have seen them in years.

"I nearly fell asleep," Fran says. "My feet feel tingly and warm, where they're usually cold." For effect, she kicks off her right pump and makes me feel the radiant foot warmth.

Marion's verdict: "I really loved it. I've had facials before, but she did a really deep massage, and the mask . . . I fell asleep at one point, but woke myself with a snort. And just touch my skin."

Fran cops a feel of her sister's newly buffed visage and promptly exclaims: "Marion, your face feels like a baby's ass!"

Recommended Treatments for Seniors

For rheumatoid arthritis in hands and feet, request a deep-heat paraffin treatment combined with a therapeutic foot soak, which motivates blood flow to help cure cold feet and smoothes skin.

Massage: either full body or focused on trouble spots such as back and neck for soothing relaxation.

Facials for skin health maintenance and skin irritations. Also a feel-good service. Manicures and pedicures are nice, too. A little polish on the toes can go a long way.

Body wraps can be modified for senior citizens who might be heat-sensitive; heat can be lessened or increased for those who get easily chilled. HealthWinds uses algae for mineralization and mud for psoriasis treatments.

Body polishes are good because they get rid of dead skin through exfoliation, help bring blood flow to the surface and aid in skin dryness problems.

Information

HealthWinds Spa. 2401 Yonge Street, Toronto, ON. Phone: (416) 488-9545.
Web: http://www.healthwindsspa.com.
The Spa at Hockley Valley Resort. On Mono 3rd Line, five kilometres north of Highway 9, northeast of Orangeville, ON. Phone: (519) 942-0754 or (416) 363-5490.
Web: http://www.hockley.com.
Spas Ontario. Web: http://www.spasontario.com.